Walk With Ease

YOUR G
BETTE
FITN

SECOND EDITION

By the *Arthritis Foundation*

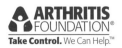

An official publication of the Arthritis Foundation
Atlanta, Georgia

Walk With Ease is a Silver Award winner in the 2000 National Health Information Awards, "honoring the nation's best consumer health information programs and materials."

An Official Publication of the Arthritis Foundation
Atlanta, Georgia

This book is not intended as a substitute for the medical advice of physicians. The reader should regularly consult a physician in matters relating to his or her health and particularly in respect of any symptoms that may require diagnosis or medical attention.

Library of Congress PCN: 2002100858

Published by
The Arthritis Foundation
1330 West Peachtree Street
Atlanta, GA 30309

Printed in Canada

The mission of the Arthritis Foundation is to improve lives through leadership in the prevention, control and cure of arthritis and related diseases.

Acknowledgments

The *Walk With Ease* program was developed by Terrie Heinrich Rizzo, MAS, Program Director, Health and Fitness Education, Stanford Health Improvement Program, Stanford Center for Research in Disease Prevention.

The information and strategies contained throughout the *Walk With Ease* program are based on research studies and tested programs in the fields of exercise science, behavior modification, and arthritis patient education. In particular, these include research and programs done by the Stanford University Arthritis Center; Kate Lorig, RN, DrPH, a nurse and expert in patient education and arthritis self-management; Albert Bandur, PhD, a social psychologist; and Marian Minor, PT, PhD, a physical therapist and expert in exercise and arthritis.

Walk With Ease was based on a pilot program developed by Donna Everix, PT, as part of the San Mateo (California) Arthritis Project (SMAP). The program was developed following the theme of "EASE" (Encourage Arthritis Support and Education).

Additional support for the development of this edition was provided by Shannon W. Mescher, M.Ed., CHES, Vice President, Programs and Services, and Linda R. Spence, MS, Director, Program Development and Resources, both of the Arthritis Foundation.

Table of Contents

Introduction

The verdict on walking is in, and it couldn't be better news. Walking is an excellent form of exercise that's good for nearly everyone, from absolute beginners to people who have been fit for years. This easy workout can help you gain all the benefits of exercise, from weight loss to stress control. Walking is easy to do and doesn't require a health club membership, fancy shoes or special training. You can do it with friends, loved ones, your pet or by yourself.

And the best news of all: Walking is safe and beneficial for most people with arthritis and other chronic conditions. So even if you have not exercised in a long time due to pain, stiffness or just feeling like you can't do it, walking may be the answer for you!

Why Walk?

Walking, like many other forms of exercise, has many fantastic benefits for the human body. Here are just a few great reasons why walking is good for your body and spirit.

Walking:
- strengthens the heart and lungs;
- nourishes joints;
- builds bones;
- fights osteoporosis, a disease marked by loss of bone mass;
- burns calories;
- helps control weight;

- reduces stress;
- boosts energy;
- is inexpensive;
- requires little previous experience;
- is convenient; and
- is fun!

If those dozen reasons aren't enough, here's the clincher: Walking is safer and puts less stress on the body than most other forms of *aerobic* exercise (the kind that builds stamina and boosts cardiovascular fitness). Walking is an especially good exercise choice if you are older or have been less active.

Most people with arthritis, a chronic condition often marked by joint pain, inflammation, stiffness and limited mobility, can walk for exercise. If you can be on your feet for about 10 minutes to do household chores, shopping or social activities, then you'll probably be able to begin a walking program to improve your health. Even if you can't stay on your feet quite that long or can only go a short distance, it's still likely that you'll be able to develop a modified walking routine that will benefit your health and help you feel better.

However, there are some people who should not walk for exercise. Consult your physician before starting this or any other exercise routine. This is especially important if you have certain serious medical conditions or symptoms. Always check with your doctor before starting anything new that might have an impact on your body, whether it's a diet, a new exercise activity, or an over-the-counter drug or supplement. Just because something seems or claims to be "healthy" doesn't mean that it will be good for *you.* So get your doctor's OK first!

Additionally, if you have arthritis-related pain that is severe and ongoing, or if you experience more than moderate discomfort in your lower extremities when you walk a very short distance, then you probably should not walk for exercise on land or other hard surfaces. Instead, consider some other type of aerobic exercise (such as water aerobics or swimming, for example) or ask your doctor or physical therapist for advice.

Unless you're in those few categories, chances are that you will be able to get going on a great walking program. For the vast majority of people with and without arthritis, this is the perfect exercise choice.

What You Can Learn From This Book

A quick note: *Walk With Ease* was written specifically for people with arthritis – but it can be a practical and useful resource for anyone, whether you have arthritis or not! The contents are based on the latest research in exercise science, plus lots of hands-on, helpful suggestions from thousands of people both with and without arthritis who have shared their experiences to help make walking work for *you.*

Whether you already walk regularly or you haven't yet started, this book will offer you many suggestions based on proven techniques concerning the right way to build and maintain a walking program. You'll learn valuable tips and strategies to improve your comfort, your safety, and your ability to "stick with it," even when you don't feel like exercising.

No matter what your current level of fitness, using this book will help you move through recognized "stages of change" to achieve the successful, long-lasting kind of program that will benefit your health and fitness level. These stages of change are:

0 - Not thinking of changing a behavior (such as walking more to improve your health)
1 - Starting to think about changing (If you're reading this book, you're at least at this stage)
2 - Clarifying your attitudes and beliefs
3 - Getting started
4 - Sticking with it
5 - Maintaining an acceptable level of activity
6 - Anticipating and overcoming problems and barriers

If you're already at Stage 5 or 6, congratulations! You are already committed. You'll probably pick up some good tips and strategies in this book for dealing with arthritis and exercise, and you can use these to help refine your personal walking program.

Most people are between Stage 0 (they haven't even started to think about getting going yet) and Stage 3 (the getting started part). Many others start exercise programs but repeatedly encounter problems at Stage 4 (sticking with it). If you're in any of these stages, you can use our program to help you develop a personal plan that works.

Walk With Ease will present many suggestions and strategies to help you move to (or remain at) Stages 5 and 6 – success and improved fitness. To get there, you will learn and practice how to:

1. Set realistic goals;
2. Develop a doable plan for implementation;
3. Learn to avoid pitfalls.

How To Use This Book

There is no "one-size-fits-all" program for successful physical activity, including walking. Everyone has different experiences and different types of obstacles to overcome, whether physical or mental. You need to determine your personal starting point on the road to better fitness and health. Your starting point is exactly where you are right now.

First, consider your mental starting point: Are you mentally ready to make walking a part of your everyday life? Are you determined to make time for your walking routine and stick with your goals so that you can achieve better health? If so, now you need to figure out your physical starting point – that is, the amount of time you currently can walk without discomfort, whether it's for one minute at a time, 10 minutes at a time, 20 minutes at a time or more.

If you currently are able to walk for at least 10 minutes, regardless of your speed, you should be able to follow our guidelines just about "as is." The information presented will help you develop a lasting personal walking routine while you deal with issues of safe exercise, pain management and motivation that affect nearly everyone.

On the other hand, if you have been inactive, have health problems other than arthritis, or have significant limitations to your hips, knees or ankles, you may not be able to walk more than a few minutes without discomfort. If so, this book can work for you, too. Just disregard any suggested time guidelines and go at your own pace. For everyone, the important thing is to *do what you can do*, and not give up activity because of discomfort, inconvenience, limitations or other difficulties.

Here are a few suggestions on how you can pick and choose parts of this book that may be of particular use to you. No matter what your starting point or personal challenges, *Walk With Ease* will have something to benefit your fitness efforts. Consider your starting level, your needs, your own style, and how you go about achieving a goal:

- If you currently are not exercising or are middle-aged or older, you should pay special attention to Chapters 1, 2 and 3.

- If you're already involved in a walking program (Stages 4 through 6 as described on page x), you're well on your way! Scan or review the information in Chapters 1 and 2, and then focus on the information in Chapters 3 through 6 to help you maintain your program.

- If you like a logical, sequential and behavioral approach to learning something, read through all the chapters in sequence. Read the information, try out the suggestions, revise if necessary and then try again.

- If factual information based on scientific research helps you understand and become motivated to do something for your health, focus on Chapters 1 and 2.

- If you think your ability to stick to an exercise program is related to outside factors, such as social or environmental challenges, pay close attention to Chapter 4.

- If lack of time is a major barrier to physical activity, check the subsections of Chapter 4.

- If pain or discomfort is a significant barrier to increasing your physical activity, see Chapter 5 as well as subsections in Chapters 1 and 3.

Everyone is different – but we all want better health. Increasing physical activity is one of the best ways to improve health, reduce pain and manage chronic conditions such as arthritis.

At the end of each chapter, we will ask you to assess your own progress through an activity called a self-check. For each self-check, ask yourself the questions, and check the box if you agree with the statement. If you are not able to check the box, go back and see how you can meet each of the goals.

Self-Check

❑ I'm at least at Stage 1, 2 or 3 on the change scale.

❑ I'm willing to budget some time to get the benefits of walking.

Remember

There is something you can actively do to reduce the limitations of arthritis.

CHAPTER 1

Starting Off Right: Know the Basic Facts About Arthritis and Exercise

Arthritis Basics

An estimated 43 million Americans are affected by more than 100 types of arthritis or related musculoskeletal conditions. One in every six people and one in three families are affected. The word "arthritis" literally means "inflammation of the joints," but that's a little misleading – not all forms of arthritis involve inflammation.

Depending on which condition you have, muscles, connective tissues, bones or other body organs may be affected. In general, arthritis and related conditions cause pain in and around joints, and make it hard to move.

What causes arthritis? Specific causes are known for some forms of arthritis but not for most. Because there are so many types of arthritis, there are likely to be many different causes.

Scientists currently are studying the roles of three major components in the cause puzzle: how you live, what happens to your body during your life and genetic factors you inherit from your parents. Of these, several specific factors appear to increase your risk for developing certain determinants of arthritis:

- People who are overweight have a higher occurrence of many kinds of arthritis, including gout (especially men) and osteoarthritis of the knees, and possibly hips. How much of a factor is excess weight? For some forms, apparently quite a lot. For example, research shows that overweight middle-age women who lose 11 pounds or more over 10 years cut their risk for developing knee arthritis in half!

- An injury that occurs to a joint or connective tissue increases risk for some types of musculoskeletal condition, such as tendinitis, bursitis, carpal tunnel syndrome and osteoarthritis of the knees and spine. These types of injuries can result from accidental damage or repetitive overuse, including sports-related injuries, accidents or job-related repetitive movements, such as repetitive deep knee-bending, lifting, reaching or typing.

- Heredity plays a significant predisposing role for certain forms of arthritis. Although arthritis is not inherited in the sense of being directly passed from parents to children, a susceptibility or tendency can be inherited for a few types. Specific forms of arthritis that are linked to heredity include rheumatoid arthritis, ankylosing spondylitis and osteoarthritis of the finger joints.

Exercise and Arthritis

The value of exercise and physical activity in improving your general health, reducing risks and fighting arthritis symptoms absolutely cannot be overstated. The benefits received from regular exercise have been documented by hundreds of studies: People who are physically active are healthier, feel better and live longer than people who are inactive. Here's why:

Regular exercise (like walking) decreases:

- Anxiety
- Blood pressure
- Blood triglycerides and glucose (sugars)
- Body fat percentage
- Bone loss
- Constipation
- Depression
- Falls and fractures
- Frailty and disability of older people
- Resting heart rate
- Risk of heart attack
- Stress

Regular exercise helps improve:

- Ability to regulate body temperature
- Aerobic capacity
- Balance
- Blood sugar tolerance
- Bone density
- Flexibility
- HDL (good) cholesterol
- Life span
- Metabolic rate
- Muscle mass
- Overall general health
- Quality of life
- Quality of sleep
- Reaction time
- Self-esteem
- Strength

But regardless of all these general health benefits, many people still believe the myth that exercise is not good for people with arthritis. They are afraid that physical activity will damage their joints and make their arthritis worse.

Wrong! Research studies (see Chapter 7) support the fact that most people with arthritis can safely get all the benefits of exercise *without* increasing damage or worsening symptoms. These studies show that for most people with arthritis, appropriate regular exercise leads to *better* flexibility, strength and endurance, and to *less* pain, fatigue and depression.

What Kinds of Exercise and How Much?

Three basic types of exercise are important for everyone, especially people with arthritis. These types are *range-of-motion* (also known as stretching or flexibility), *muscle-strengthening* and *aerobic* (also known as endurance) exercises. Each plays a role in improving your overall health and fitness, as well as reducing arthritis-related disability and pain.

Range-of-Motion and Stretching (Flexibility) Exercises

Daily stretching activities counteract one of the most devastating consequences of arthritis: the decreased ability to move your joints through their fullest degrees of movement, called range of motion (ROM).

Losing ROM translates into less ability to do the basic, everyday activities of daily living (for example, simple things like reaching up to kitchen cabinets or bending down to pick up something off the floor). Maintaining ROM is crucial for your quality of life, so flexibility exercises are the foundation of most therapeutic exercise programs for people with arthritis.

To keep joints mobile and to improve function, flexibility exercises should be done gently and smoothly for 10 to 15 minutes a day, usually every day. Flexibility exercises also are important to do before and after recreational or fitness activities, because stretched muscles and joints help you maintain balance, avoid falls and prevent injuries. You should do a few easy but important stretches before and after you walk, as will be described more fully in Chapter 3.

If you have been inactive for some time, or have pain or stiffness that interferes with daily activities, start your exercise program by building a routine of general flexibility exercises. For suggested exercises, talk with your doctor or therapist, or consult *The Arthritis Foundation's Guide to Managing Your Arthritis*. When you can do 10 minutes of continuous flexibility movements daily, you will have the motion and endurance needed to include muscle-strengthening exercises and aerobic activity into your program.

Another great source of exercise guidance for you if you have arthritis and have not exercised in a while is PACE – People with Arthritis Can Exercise. This program, offered by the Arthritis Foundation, can be taken in a class format (by calling your local chapter of the Arthritis Foundation – see the Resources section at the end of this book) or at home using one of the PACE videos appropriate for your fitness level.

Muscle-Strengthening Exercises

Muscle strength is important for two reasons. One, stronger muscles help provide support to joints affected by arthritis. Two, stronger muscles help you maintain the functional strength necessary to perform everyday tasks (for example, climbing stairs, working in the garden or picking up bags of groceries).

Strengthening exercises need only be done three to four times a week and not on consecutive days unless advised otherwise by your doctor. There are two main kinds of strengthening exercises:

- **Isometric exercises** – isometrics involve tightening muscles with minimal movement of the joints or limbs. You do this either by tensing one set of muscles against another (for example, pressing the front of one leg against the back of the other) or by tensing a set of muscles against an immovable object (for example, pushing your arm against the wall).

- **Isotonic exercises** – isotonics involve the movement of a joint or limb against some kind of resistance. Resisting against gravity (for example, raising your leg up and down) or against weights (for example, lifting light weights or food cans to shoulder height) are both forms of isotonic exercise. Isotonic exercises develop strength throughout the muscle's full range of motion and generally result in greater overall strength gains.

If your arthritis is not particularly limiting, you probably can do basic strengthening exercises safely by following recommended rules for proper techniques and safety. Especially remember to start slowly and avoid doing too much, too soon. For suggested exercises, call the Arthritis Foundation at 800/283-7800 for materials, log on to the Arthritis Foundation Web site, **www. arthritis.org**, consult *Managing Your Arthritis* or talk to your doctor or physical therapist.

However, if you are older, if you have been very inactive, or if you have rheumatoid arthritis or another condition with limitations, it is important that your strength program be carefully designed for your specific needs. Knowing which muscles need to be strengthened and how to perform the exercises without stressing your joints are key elements in a successful program. Do not engage in strengthening exercises before talking to your doctor or physical therapist for appropriate recommendations.

Aerobic (Endurance) Exercises

Aerobic exercise is the kind that strengthens your heart, lungs and blood vessels, and gives you more stamina so you can do more with less effort. Aerobic exercise also relieves pain and stiffness by improving blood circulation throughout your body and by releasing a set of hormones called endorphins, which actually diminish the perception of pain.

To be aerobic, exercise needs to involve the continuous, rhythmic movement of your large muscles (your largest ones are in your legs, buttocks and upper back/shoulders) and last long enough to raise and sustain your heart rate. Walking is one of the best forms of aerobic exercise for people with arthritis. Others are swimming, aquatics, cycling, low-impact aerobic dancing and exercising on equipment such as treadmills, ski machines or stationary bicycles.

Daily activities such as raking leaves, walking the dog, mowing the lawn or going out dancing also can count as aerobic activities. Note that all of these involve sustained, repetitive movements of your large muscles. Jogging and running also are aerobic, but these produce more strain on the joints.

Contrary to what many people think, aerobic exercise does not have to be really strenuous, unless that's what you want to do! Good news from recent research is that moderate physical activity produces the same health benefits as strenuous activities do, with far less risk of injury. What's moderate? Here's a good rule of thumb: At a moderate level, you should feel as if your body is working, but you should still be able to talk fairly normally and carry on at a comfortable pace. To get the health benefits of physical activity, current recommendations are for 30 minutes of moderate activity on most days of the week. Your minimum goal should be at least 120-150 minutes of moderate physical activity each week.

That may sound like a lot, especially in the beginning – but don't worry. The idea is to do what you can do now, and build gradually.

Our walking plan is designed to help you build up to 30-minute (or longer) sessions on three to five days per week. However, even if you never are able to do all 30 minutes at a time, don't worry. The second important news from recent research is that your 30 minutes of moderate physical activity can be accumulated in three 10-minute bouts over the course of the day for the same health benefits as one continuous 30-minute session.

This book will help you build your program to the longest segments that are manageable for you. For example, to get your total of 30 minutes, you could rake leaves for 10 minutes, later take a 10-minute walk, and then wash your car for 10 minutes.

But What If Exercise Hurts?

It's important to recognize right here at the beginning that exercising may not be pain-free. For many people with arthritis, exercise can be accompanied by temporary discomfort and new feelings in your muscles and around your joints. You may experience any of the following: some cramping or fatigue in your muscles while you walk, knee discomfort during or after walking, soreness around your ankles, and muscle soreness in your calves and thighs after walking.

If you have a little discomfort that you can bear as you make the transition into your walking program, that's OK – it may not be fun, but rest assured, it's not harmful. Try walking more slowly, make sure you are wearing supportive shoes, and only walk on level surfaces. Do everything you can to manage pain by following the tips in Chapter 5, but don't give up on walking because of temporary discomfort.

Use the Two-Hour Pain Rule as a Guideline

If you have more pain two hours after you finish walking than before you started, then you have overdone it. Cut back until you find a level that does not cause more pain two hours after you finish than you had before you started.

This rule makes sense for everyone – and you'll be reminded of the two-hour pain rule many times throughout this book. Always keep in mind that you are not causing damage to yourself – and remind yourself of all the health benefits you are gaining. If you have increased, lasting or severe pain in hips or knees when you walk, talk to your doctor or therapist.

To summarize, the evidence concerning exercise and arthritis is loud and clear:

- Your overall program should include three basic kinds of exercise: flexibility, strengthening and aerobic activity.

- You will not cause damage to yourself with appropriate exercise.

- You *can* cause damage to yourself by NOT exercising!

Exercise Dos and Don'ts

Here are some general principles to follow to keep exercise as safe and pain-free as possible.

DO:

✓ Build a program that includes three different kinds of exercise: range-of-motion, strengthening exercises and aerobic exercise.

✓ Walk when you have the least pain and stiffness.

✓ Walk when you are not tired.

✓ Walk when your medicine (if you are taking any) is having its greatest effect.

✓ Always include a warm-up and a cool-down (discussed in Chapter 3) whenever you walk.

✓ Start at your own ability level, move slowly and gently, and progress gradually.

✓ Avoid becoming chilled or overheated when walking.

✓ Use heat, cold and other strategies to minimize pain. (The following chapters will include many pain-management tips.)

✓ Use aids, like walking sticks or canes, if they help.

✓ Expect that walking may cause some discomfort. (But not too much! See "Don'ts" on the opposite page.)

DON'T:

✗ Do too much, too soon. Start slowly and gradually.

✗ Hold your breath when doing anything! Remember, keep breathing.

✗ Take extra medicine before walking to relieve or prevent joint or muscle pain unless prescribed by your doctor.

✗ Don't walk so fast or far that you have more pain two hours after you finish than before you started (the two-hour pain rule).

Additional Information for Specific Conditions

Osteoarthritis (OA)

Osteoarthritis is the most common form of arthritis and now affects more than 21 million Americans. This number is expected to grow significantly as the "baby boomer" population ages. Also sometimes known as degenerative joint disease (DJD), OA is characterized by gradual, degenerative wear-and-tear of joint cartilage, which usually affects only a few specific joints rather than appearing throughout the body.

OA commonly affects the knees and other weight-bearing joints such as the hips and lower back. Other common sites include the neck, ankles, thumbs and the finger joints.

Severity of OA varies from person to person; joint discomfort can range from mild to severe. The majority of people with OA will not experience severe disability, crippling or joint misalignments, and most can manage OA by using a variety of strategies, including medicines and pain-management techniques. Recent advances in joint replacement have been beneficial for people with severe OA of the hips or knees.

What about exercise for people with OA? Years ago, people with OA were advised to stay off affected joints – but not anymore. Treatment for OA now emphasizes the importance of exercise. We now know that cartilage needs joint motion to stay healthy. The motion of exercise both delivers nourishment to the joints and gets rid of waste products. Without motion, this vital exchange cannot take place. Joint cartilage actually deteriorates if a joint is not moved regularly.

If you have OA, follow the general exercise dos and don'ts listed on pages 12 & 13. Additionally, keep these points in mind:

- Remember that all joints, especially those with OA, need to be moved regularly and taken through their full range of motion several times daily to maintain flexibility and take care of cartilage. Observe safety precautions, but avoid babying joints with OA.

- However, just as too much rest is bad for joints with OA, so is too much activity. If joints are continually compressed (as the hips and knees are by long periods of standing) the cartilage can't expand and soak up nutrients and fluid. Therefore, it is important to avoid long periods of compression, and to alternate activity and rest throughout the day.

- It is very important for you to strike a balance between getting enough exercise and getting enough rest. How much is too much? Follow the two-hour pain rule: Your goal is to exercise so that pain is not worse two hours after you exercise than before you started. If you do too much, cut back the next time to a point that is comfortable. Adjust until you find a level that works for you.

- If you have OA in your hips or knees, avoid types of exercise that overload these joints, such as climbing or very fast walking. Also, be sure to follow exercise with at least an hour off your feet to give cartilage time to decompress.

- If you have had a joint replaced, consult your doctor before attempting any stretching or strengthening exercises for that part of your body. When engaging in aerobic exercise like walking, remember that certain precautions apply to artificial hips and knees, and you need to respect these if you want the joint to last as long as possible.

- Always practice good posture and wear supportive shoes. Both of these will help protect cartilage and reduce joint pain. (Chapter 2 will provide additional information about shoes and good posture.)

- Be sure to do strengthening exercises. Toned muscles with good endurance help support joints. Key muscle groups to strengthen generally include the muscles that help support the hips, knees and ankles. (See recommended exercises in Appendix A.) Other muscle groups to include in your overall strengthening program are those that support the hands, wrists, elbows and back. (These exercises are not included in this book. Talk to your therapist or consult the Arthritis Foundation for recommended exercises.)

- It is critical for you to keep your body weight under control. Excess weight accelerates damage to weight-bearing joints. Even ten or twenty extra pounds multiplies the force absorbed by your feet, knees, hips and back – not only when you're exercising, but also when you're just going about your daily activities!

Rheumatoid Arthritis (RA)

Rheumatoid arthritis is the condition that many people think of when they hear the word arthritis. RA is a systemic (meaning that it may affect the whole body), autoimmune disease in which the immune system attacks the body's own tissues, causing an inflammation of the lining of the joints and/or other internal organs.

RA typically affects many different joints throughout

the body, usually symmetrically; that is, similarly on both sides of the body. (This is very different from OA, which usually affects only a few specific joints and often is one-sided.) Joints that may be affected by RA include the hands (except for the joints closest to the fingernails), thumbs, wrists, elbows, shoulders, neck and jaw, as well as the hips, knees, ankles and feet.

Along with joint problems, RA can cause generalized fatigue, decreased appetite and weight loss. With RA, it is typical to see periods of inflammation, called exacerbations or flares, followed by remissions, which vary from individual to individual. Symptoms of a flare can include joint swelling, redness, warmth, pain, tenderness, fatigue, morning stiffness, muscle aches and a feeling of being sick.

It is very important for people with RA to achieve the proper balance between exercise and rest, especially during flares. When a joint is hot, painful and swollen, resting helps reduce inflammation, which is good – but with too much rest, muscles lose strength, ligaments and tendons become less strong and bones get softer. Even in healthy young men, research shows that three weeks of lying in bed can reduce fitness as much as 30 years of normal aging does – and just one week of immobility can cause a muscle to lose up to 30 percent of its mass! Immobility also greatly increases your risk of developing osteoporosis. It is important that you learn how to adjust your activities to achieve the best physical health.

If you have RA, keep these points in mind:

- When you have flares, rest as needed, but remember that rest does not mean stopping all activities. Be sure to continue doing very gentle movements. These should include gentle range-of-motion exercises to help maintain joint mobility. Your doctor or physical therapist can guide you.

- Aquatic exercise can usually be continued during flares, since the buoyancy of the water helps support joints, making movement easier.

- During non-flare periods when symptoms are under control, doing low-impact weight-bearing activity like walking is important for your overall health. Discuss specific recommendations with your doctor or therapist, including any restrictions or modifications for your particular condition. Whenever you have flares, cut back as necessary but gradually work back up to a full program again as soon as you can.

- Additionally, during non-flare periods you should do regular flexibility and strengthening exercises to maintain the range of motion and strength of supporting muscles necessary for everyday activities. It is important that your flexibility and strength exercises be carefully designed for your specific needs. Knowing which muscles need to be strengthened and how to perform the exercises without stressing your joints is important. Do not engage in strengthening exercises before talking to your doctor or physical therapist about appropriate recommendations.

- Always be sure to pay careful attention to using your joints appropriately when exercising. Maintaining good posture and joint motion during exercise helps ease joint pain and avoid tightness.

- You may not feel like exercising, especially during flares. Remember that movement is important for you to prevent loss of mobility – be sure your exercise is appropriate, and be sure to do it!

Fibromyalgia

Fibromyalgia is another common arthritis-related condition. Is is not actually a joint condition, but instead is a form of soft-tissue or muscular rheumatism – the name fibromyalgia means pain in the muscles and fibrous connective tissues (the ligaments and tendons).

Fibromyalgia is characterized by pain and aching in many parts of the body. Symptoms include moderate to severe fatigue, lack of energy, decreased exercise endurance, sleep disturbances, headaches, widespread muscle aches and "tender points" in specific body locations. Other symptoms can include tingling in the face or extremities (hands, arms, feet or legs), abdominal pain or bloating, alternating constipation and diarrhea, urinary urgency and skin sensitivity. Fibromyalgia pain often varies according to time of day, activity level, sleep patterns, stress and weather. Most people with fibromyalgia say that some degree of pain is always present, and often the aches and discomfort feel like a persistent flu.

Exercise for this condition is still being investigated, but it now appears that one of the major principles of treatment is aerobic exercise that is slowly increased toward full cardiovascular conditioning and physical fitness. However, because muscles usually are tight, sore and very vulnerable to decreased circulation and minor injury, it is important to observe several specific principles when doing your needed exercise.

If you have fibromyalgia, here are points to remember:

- A specific combination of exercise can be an important part of your treatment program by helping you reduce muscle tension, decrease pain and aid relaxation. This combination includes: 1) regularly participating in low-intensity aerobic activity to improve conditioning and maintain good circulation (all great reasons to walk!); 2) carefully performing stretching exercises before and after your aerobic activity to reduce the likelihood of muscle or joint strains and to maintain good range of motion; and 3) carefully observing safety recommendations for exercise in general – especially if you are doing strengthening exercises – to avoid the possibility of minor injuries such as muscle pulls or joint strains.

- Be aware that fibromyalgia symptoms often get worse, not better, with vigorous exercise – so it is important that you always start slowly, do only low- to moderate-intensity exercise, and avoid fast movements or high impact.

- You may not feel like exercising when you are tired or in pain. Remember that exercise is an important part of your treatment. See Chapters 4 and 5 for strategies to help manage pain and stay motivated.

The Arthritis Foundation has a new series of books, *Good Living*, designed to help people with osteoarthritis, rheumatoid arthritis and fibromyalgia. Each book focuses on the specific disease, offering clear explanations of causes and symptoms, diagnostic tests, drugs and surgical therapies, alternative therapies and self-management techniques, including detailed stretching exercises. Learn more about these and other Arthritis Foundation books in the Resources section at the end of this book.

Osteoporosis

Osteoporosis is a bone disorder in which the bones lose density, become thin and weak, and break more easily. Although anyone can have osteoporosis, it is most common in older people, particularly women who are past menopause. The National Osteoporosis Foundation estimates that more than 28 million Americans, most of whom are women, have osteoporosis or are at high-risk for developing osteoporosis.

Osteoporosis contributes to compression fractures of the spine (fractures in which the spinal vertebrae become flattened), resulting in significant pain and loss of height. Multiple fractures often cause a height loss of four or more inches and result in a curved spine that is sometimes called a dowager's hump or widow's hump. (The correct term for this forward curvature is kyphosis.) With osteoporosis, common movements like lifting, bending over or even moving the wrong way in bed can result in spinal compression fractures and severe pain.

Bones that are fragile from osteoporosis break easily in falls or accidents. As a direct result of osteoporosis, one in five women breaks a hip before the age of 75. Wrist fractures resulting from falls occur in more than 250,000 women each year, and fractures of the pelvis, ankle, ribs and shoulder also frequently occur.

Exercise is an extraordinarily important part in both osteoporosis prevention and treatment programs. In particular, weight-bearing exercise such as walking or jogging (where your body weight bears down on your feet as you stand, requiring your bones to support the weight of your body against gravity) plays one of the most significant roles in preventing osteoporosis from developing if started in earlier years – or in retarding further loss of bone density once osteoporosis has developed. One of the best forms of weight-bearing exercise is walking.

If you have osteoporosis, here are points to remember:

- If you have had a hip fracture, you must discuss any proposed exercise program with your doctor first, to be sure the movements are appropriate for you.

- If you have had a spinal fracture that has occurred in the last 6 months, it is desirable for you to start exercising as soon as your pain will permit. (Check with your doctor if you have questions.) You may have to go a little slower than a woman who is at risk for fracture but hasn't had one – nevertheless, begin as soon as you can. Remember, bone loss – which increases your risk of having additional fractures – is accelerated by inactivity and bed rest.

- Walking for 20 to 60 minutes, three to five times a week, is recommended to help maintain bone strength. If 20 to 60 minutes in one session is too much for you, smaller segments are fine. Your goal should be to try to accumulate a total of at least 90 to 120 minutes each week of moving on your feet, in the longest time periods you can manage. This can be done in lots of ways. For example, to total 120 minutes you can take six 20-minute walks weekly (one walk per day), 12 10-minute walks weekly (two per day) or 24 five-minute walks weekly (four per day).

- General stretching and strength-training exercises are important to help maintain posture and to support your spine. Special emphasis should be placed on exercises that strengthen the hips, thighs, back, arms and shoulders. For recommended exercises, check with your physical therapist or an exercise instructor who is knowledgeable about osteoporosis, or ask your doctor. (Also see the Resources list in Chapter 7.)

- Don't perform any exercise or activity that requires you to bend forward at the waist or mid-back with your back rounded (this is called spinal flexion). This posture dramatically increases the forces on your spine. This means no sit-ups, no abdominal crunches, toe-touches or use of exercise equipment that require this position. There are safer alternatives for exercising all of these muscle groups, including your abdominals. Again, check with your physical therapist or a qualified exercise instructor.

- Don't perform any exercise or activity that requires you to move your leg sideways or across your body, especially against resistance (this is called abduction or adduction of the leg). This kind of movement usually occurs with certain specific exercises or resistance-exercise machines. A hip weakened by osteoporosis may be more susceptible to breaking when stressed in this manner.

- Whether walking for exercise or going about everyday activities, avoid jarring your spine. This action increases your risk of spinal compression fractures. Be especially careful to avoid activities that make falls more likely. Don't walk on slippery floors or surfaces, and avoid wearing hard, smooth-soled shoes. Be particularly careful when walking on uneven surfaces or icy sidewalks. If your balance is poor, if you feel awkward or if you are doing any motions that involve twisting or bending, use a walking stick or cane for support.

Other Forms of Arthritis and Related Conditions

Other conditions in the general family of arthritis and related rheumatic disorders include gout, ankylosing spondylitis, systemic lupus erythematosus (lupus), polymyalgia rheumatica, bursitis, tendinitis, carpal tunnel syndrome, scleroderma, Raynaud's phenomenon and psoriatic arthritis, among many others. For information about these or the many other forms of arthritis, talk with your doctor or contact the Arthritis Foundation.

Conditions Requiring Supervised Exercise

Most people can walk for exercise with little problem. However for some people, aerobic exercise like walking may be risky or possible only under special supervised conditions (that is, an exercise session during which a doctor or other qualified health professional is present or overseeing the exercise).

If you have any of the following conditions – or if you are not sure – check with your doctor before you start any exercise program on your own, including walking:

- History of joint surgery due to arthritis

- Arthritis or related condition in which the heart, lungs, blood vessels or nervous system is involved

- Another disease or condition that makes aerobic exercise problematic because it may cause exercise-related complications, such as:

  - chronic bronchitis or emphysema
  - coronary artery or heart disease
  - peripheral vascular disease
  - diabetes
  - cancer
  - extreme obesity

- A physical condition or disease known to limit or prevent any unsupervised exercise, such as:

  - acute or inadequately controlled heart failure
  - unstable angina pectoris or a recent severe heart attack
  - uncontrolled arrhythmias (irregular heart beats)
  - a recent embolism
  - thrombophlebitis
  - moderate to severe aortic stenosis
  - resting heart rate greater than 120 beats per minute
  - uncontrolled hypertension (with resting systolic blood pressure above 200 mmHg or diastolic blood pressure above 120 mmHg)
  - uncontrolled metabolic disease (such as diabetes mellitus or myxedema)

- fever (oral temperature of 99.5 or above)
- acute infection
- chronic infectious disease (such as hepatitis or AIDS)
- any other condition known to preclude exercise

If you are not sure, check with your doctor! Your doctor is the best source of information for you if you have genuine concerns about how you should exercise.

Note that several of these symptoms – including fever and acute infections – often are temporary and affect nearly everyone. If you have these symptoms, stop walking until you feel better. It's always better to err on the side of caution!

Further Questions About Exercise or Modifications

If you have additional questions related to exercise or modifications for your form of arthritis or related condition, talk with your doctor or physical therapist. Take this book along and discuss with him or her what you should do. Be sure to discuss the best level of intensity and time duration for your walks (these are described more fully in Chapter 2). Also, talk about modifications or special needs you may have. With adaptations as needed, most people with arthritis can develop a successful exercise program that includes walking.

Self-Check

❏ I know the basic facts about arthritis and exercise.

❏ I believe that I would feel better if I increased my exercise by walking regularly.

❏ I am confident I can apply the general tips about exercise and arthritis to my exercise program.

❏ I know about any specific adaptations I should observe for my form of arthritis.

❏ I know the three main types of exercise and how often I should be doing them.

Remember

The many benefits of exercise can be yours! By taking necessary precautions or making modifications to fit your special needs, you can walk for better health and well-being.

CHAPTER 2

Getting Ready and Set To Go: Preparing To *Walk With Ease*

Walking for exercise isn't complicated: You start a walking program by starting to walk! However, if you're like most people who begin an exercise program, starting is only half the battle. Good intentions usually aren't enough to keep people going for long.

After just six months, nearly half of all those who start exercising have dropped out – and another third will have quit by the end of the first year! Real long-term success almost always takes more than simply having good intentions; it takes some knowledge of basic exercise information, some preliminary preparation – and a plan.

Getting Ready:
Prepare Your Walking Equipment

One of the greatest things about walking is that you don't need a lot of equipment. All you really need are:

- The right pair of shoes for good support

- Comfortable exercise clothing

Here are some other equipment suggestions to consider acquiring:

- Watch with second hand, stopwatch or pedometer

- Walking stick or cane for balance and joint support

- Fanny pack or small purse to carry miscellaneous items like keys, identification, pocket change and a plastic water bottle if desired

Walking Shoes

Well-fitting, comfortable shoes are crucial for walking. Because the biomechanics (efficient body movements) of walking are different than those for other activities, you shouldn't use any old athletic-type shoes you happen to have around. To provide the best support and help prevent injuries, you should get a good pair of shoes made specifically for *walking*.

What's good when it comes to walking shoes? Consumers Union (publishers of *Consumer Reports*) and other groups do annual evaluations of walking shoes. These can give you some good ideas – but use those ratings only as a guide! Every shoe and every foot are different.

The best thing is to go to a specialty athletic footwear store or shoe store and try on shoes. A good store will let you take a jaunt down the sidewalk or hall, and its staff will watch you move to see if the shoe is right for you. Take the time to talk to the salesperson about the best shoe for you.

Consider the following points when evaluating a walking shoe:

- **Sole:** The shoe bottom should be made in a pattern that will grip the surface and provide traction. Avoid sticky, non-skid soles and heavy rubber lugs (ridges) that curl over the top of the toe area; these can cause tripping and falling, especially on carpets. Also avoid slick, smooth-soled shoes that make slipping and falling more likely. The store's sales professional will be able to help you choose a shoe with the proper sole for your needs.

- **Flexion:** The shoe should not be too rigid, but needs to be firm in the right place. To test for this quality, hold a shoe by the heel and toe, and bend the toe up and back: the sole of the shoe should be flexible and bend easily at the forefoot, but have a fairly firm midsole.

- **Breathability:** The upper portion of the shoe should be made of material that allows moisture to escape, so your feet stay drier. All-leather shoes or shoes with breathable mesh uppers are good choices.

- **Cushioning:** The heel area needs to provide good cushioning to absorb the impact when your heel comes down on the floor or street. Heel cushioning is very important for shock absorption for your whole body (as compared with runners who land harder on the middle of the foot – that's why running shoes aren't great for walking).

- **Support:** Rear-foot support and stability along with good arch support will help limit inward roll (pronation) while walking. If you aren't sure if the shoe provides this, check with a sales professional.

- **Proper fit:** Always try on both shoes with the same type of socks you will be wearing when walking. If you use any orthotic supports, fit them in the shoes before deciding. Shoes should fit you comfortably, have a snug heel fit so your heel doesn't slip, and have a roomy toe box – that is, the toe area should provide enough room to allow your toes to spread out. There should be a thumb's width between the end of your longest toe and the end of the shoe. Shop for shoes at the end of the day, when your feet tend to be at their largest size.

- **Closures:** Shoes with laces let you adjust as needed and give more support than slip-on shoes. If you have problems tying laces, consider *Velcro* closures or elastic shoelaces.

- **Extra cushioning and support:** Replacement insoles can be purchased from athletic or shoe stores to provide extra cushioning and support in your walking shoes. Good replacement insoles have a pre-formed heel cup and arch support that can help improve fit and stabilize your foot. Insoles come in sizes and can be trimmed with scissors for a final fit.

- **Beveled heel:** A bevel or angle in the heel of your walking shoe will permit you to achieve a smooth, rolling motion when you walk. A heel with no bevel will cause your toes to "slap" down rapidly, possibly leading to shin splints.

Don't be in a hurry when buying your walking shoes. You may have to shop around, and sacrifice color or style to get a good fit. Talk to the trained sales personnel in fitness or shoe shops, take a test walk or stand around in the shoes for a while before you decide to buy them. Your shoes should provide good support, be comfortable and your feet shouldn't hurt. Don't think that the most expensive shoe is the best one for you. Compare prices and do a little research to find the right pair.

When should you replace shoes? Probably sooner than you think – most people wait too long. Shoes might look great from the outside for years, but the insides will lose at least a third of their ability to support and absorb shock and the soles will begin to deteriorate after about 500 miles to 600 miles of walking. (That's not as much as it might seem. For example, a walker who takes 30-minute walks three times a week will need replacement shoes after about nine to 12 months.) And the insoles probably will need replacement even sooner, usually every couple of months for people who walk regularly – this is important for shock absorption. Don't continue to wear shoes or insoles when they're worn out – your body will absorb the negative effects.

Socks

Next to your shoes, socks are your feet's best friend. Having the right socks will keep your feet cool and dry, as well as properly cushioned when you walk. As with shoes, don't wear just any socks when you walk or do any other form of exercise. It's important to use socks meant for exercise. Here are a few things to know about good walking socks:

- Many walkers prefer padded socks made from a blend of acrylic fiber and cotton or wool. The acrylic wicks away perspiration from your skin, and the cotton or wool then absorbs it, so your feet stay drier and more comfortable.

- Look for snug-fitting socks with as few seams to chafe as possible.

- For some blister-prone people, wearing two pairs of socks can eliminate rubbing.

- If your socks wear through in the toes, the problem is your shoes. Either the shoes are too short, or your foot is sliding forward with each step.

- As noted above, take your walking socks when you go to purchase your shoes to help get a better fit.

Clothes

With the right clothes, you should be able to walk all seasons of the year. Clothes should be comfortable, simple and efficient. Choices range from simple loose-fitting T-shirts and shorts or sweat suits, to stretch-type walking shorts and tights. Dress as warmly as necessary for the weather.

- Clothing should allow you to move through the full range of your walking stride without binding, restricting movement or pulling.

- Pants or shorts should fit comfortably in the waist and not bind in the leg or crotch.

- Clothing made of cotton is always comfortable and absorbs perspiration. Garments with *Supplex*, polypropylene and fleece are lightweight, wick moisture away from your skin and provide insulation against the wind. Most sporting goods stores have a good choice of shorts, pants and jackets in these fabrics.

- Women should wear a comfortable bra that provides good support or a sports bra. (If you've never worn a sports bra, try one – you might like the support!)

- Always wear reflective clothing or a vest with reflectors when you are walking outdoors – even in daylight hours – so oncoming cars and trucks can see you.

- The most efficient way to maintain a comfortable body temperature is by wearing layers of clothing. Layering clothes stabilizes body temperature by trapping air between layers that can be warmed by your body heat. Layers can be removed one by one if you get too warm. It is better to start out with too many clothes and remove layers as you go, than to be underdressed and too cool to continue walking. Three layers are generally recommended:

a) The inner layer allows for absorption of moisture from the skin and, depending on the material, may pass moisture on to the next layer. Women should always wear a cotton-blend bra, which is usually enough of an inner layer during warmer months. In colder weather, particularly for outdoor walking, both women and men should choose a short- or long-sleeved T-shirt as an inner layer. On the lower body, wear cotton or nylon briefs in the warmer months, plus long underwear or tights for cold-weather outdoor walks.

b) The middle layer provides warmth and some protection from wind and cold. For the upper body, a short-sleeved T-shirt will be enough in warmer months; in cooler weather, a long-sleeved T-shirt or turtleneck is a good choice. For the lower body, shorts are usually fine if the weather is warm and there is little or no wind. Wear long pants or sweatpants if it is windy or cold.

c) An outer layer is necessary when walking in colder weather. It should be resistant to wind and rain, allow sweat to evaporate, and, in coldest temperatures, trap air to keep you warm. Nylon is a good material to wear for this layer. A zip or pullover jacket (with or without a hood) will provide protection and also is lightweight. In the coldest months, a hat (and possibly a face mask) should be worn to maintain body heat and protect your face against wind and cold. Mittens or gloves should be worn to keep hands warm.

Other Comfort Tips

- Wear a hat or visor on sunny days to protect your face from the sun.

- Keep hair away from your face; tie it back out of the way if it's long.

- Sun protection is important. Put sunscreen on all exposed body parts (don't forget neck and ears). Sunglasses reduce eyestrain and eye damage.

Getting Set:
Planning Your Program of F.I.T. Exercise

As you build a successful walking program, you'll follow the F.I.T. guidelines that are recommended by exercise experts for becoming fitter, healthier and more pain-free.

F.I.T. stands for your exercise Frequency (how often), Intensity (how hard), and Time duration (how long).

Here are the recommendations:

F= frequency

New guidelines for good health recommend some kind of moderate level physical activity on most days of the week. A good walking program would be to walk at least 3-5 days per week, and perhaps do other physical activities on other days. If you choose, walking more often is fine, up to all seven days per week – especially if you are walking for short time segments.

When you are able to go for walks of 30 minutes or longer, taking days off gives your body a chance to rest and adapt. Try to space your sessions throughout the week.

For example, if you're a four-day-a-week exerciser, you might schedule your walks for Monday, Wednesday, Friday and Sunday, rather than Monday, Tuesday, Wednesday and Thursday, followed by three straight days off.

If you walk five days per week, schedule a day off every two or three days – for example, you might walk on Tuesday, Wednesday, Thursday, Saturday and Sunday.

On non-walking days, continue to do your flexibility exercises. You should work in strengthening exercises three to four times a week.

I= intensity

Intensity refers to how much you are exerting yourself – that is, how hard you are working. The new guidelines for physical activity like walking recommend exertion at low-to-moderate intensity. What does "low-to-moderate" mean? Use your body's effort as a guideline: At low-to-moderate intensity, you will be working hard enough to feel some changes in your body, such as increased breathing, heart rate or muscle use – but not so hard that you become out of breath or feel that it's hard to keep up.

If exercise is too high in intensity (what you'd describe as hard to very hard), it most likely is too fast or too challenging for your level of fitness right now. Too-high intensity exercise almost always causes discomfort and certainly increases your risk of injury – and you're much more likely to end up dropping out.

Measuring your intensity as you exercise helps you monitor yourself for safety, so that you don't overexert. It also helps you keep track of your progress from week to week. Doing this isn't complicated. There are several easy ways to measure intensity – for example, by giving yourself a "talk test" while you're exercising, or judging how hard you are working on a scale of 1-10. For most people these informal measures work just fine, especially in the beginning. Taking your pulse is another way to measure yourself. Chapter 6 provides complete guidelines on all these techniques.

T= time duration

How much time should you spend walking? The new guidelines recommend about 30 minutes of aerobic activity on most days – that's only 120 to 180 minutes of walking out of an entire week! If 30-minute durations at a time are too much for you to start with, remember that your 30 minutes don't have to be done all at once to achieve health benefits, especially in the beginning. To get 30 minutes of activity on your exercise days, you could walk:

- 30 minutes all at once

- 10 minutes three times a day

- 5 minutes six times a day

The goal of aerobic activity like walking is to gradually build your endurance and ability to go for longer time durations. Begin slowly with short distances or take several short walks a day until you can build up to longer distances and periods of time. The walking program outlined in Chapter 3 is set up to help you.

As a long-term goal, this walking program will help you build up to 30 to 45 minutes a session on four or five days a week. However, if pain is a problem, it's OK to stay with shorter segments. You should do the most you comfortably can – your goal is 120 to 180 minutes a week, in the longest time segments you are able to do.

A Note About Impact

Impact refers to how hard your body is coming down on your feet and joints. Impact is a major consideration for many people who have arthritis, particularly cases involving the hips or knees.

In general, activities that involve a lot of impact should be avoided. Lower-impact activities (where you come down lightly on hips, knees and feet) minimize stress to joints and cause less discomfort.

To keep impact as low as possible, you can:

- Choose a form of exercise that is low-impact to begin with (like walking or aquatic exercises);

- Wear good shoes and insoles that absorb shock;

- Keep your weight at a healthy level;

- Use a walking stick or cane to help provide support for your body;

- Walk on an appropriate level surface.

What does the surface have to do with it? Actually, the surface on which you walk affects your intensity (how hard you work) the impact (how hard your body is coming down on your feet and joints) and your balance. When planning your walks, try to choose a surface level that is suitable for your ability. Some guidelines follow on the next page:

LEVEL I: Flat, firm surfaces such as school tracks, streets with sidewalks, shopping malls, fitness trails or quiet neighborhoods. Most people with arthritis and related conditions should walk on Level I surfaces.

- most adaptable for intensity (i.e., exertion from low to high intensity is possible)

- least impact to knees and hips

- least challenging to balance

LEVEL II: Some inclines or stairs, somewhat uneven ground, sand, gravel or soft earth.

- more challenging in intensity (i.e., the lowest level of exertion is harder)

- greater impact to knees and hips

- more challenging to balance

LEVEL III: Hills, very uneven ground, very loose gravel or stones, or lots of stairs. Most people with arthritis should avoid Level III surfaces when walking as an aerobic activity.

- most challenging in intensity (i.e., the lowest level of exertion is even harder)

- greatest impact to knees and hips

- most difficult for balance

Reminder: if you still cannot walk even very short distances without significant joint discomfort in your lower extremities – even after following all precautions and using appropriate pain-management strategies – then you probably should choose a non-impact form of aerobic exercise. This means a form of exercise where there is no or minimal stress placed on your hips, knees and feet, such as swimming or aquatics.

Developing Your Walking Plan

Research shows that one of the best ways to help you succeed is to actually make a written plan. An easy-to-do sample plan is included below. Make a copy, or develop your own play with features you like. Follow these steps:

Step 1: Make a Contract With Yourself

Decide how long you will commit to this program. Six to 10 weeks is a reasonable time commitment for a new program.

Then, make a specific plan. This is the hardest and most important part of your contract with yourself. This must be something that 1) you feel you realistically can do, and 2) is an achievable step on the way to your long-term goals. For example, many people can't start off by walking for 30 minutes (long-term goal) – but most people can walk for at least a few minutes to begin with (achievable step).

Keep in mind that what you plan will depend on the level of your exercise readiness. For example:

- If you have been extremely limited in your activities because of pain or disability, your first goal may be to walk five minutes at a time in your own home or around the block each day.

- If you have fallen into inactivity by habit or discomfort, you may be able to start out by walking – slowly – for 10 minutes at a time, three times a week.

- If you're already active, you may be able to go for longer walks, perhaps for 20 minutes or more at a time, three to six times a week.

Your personal contract plan should contain the following steps. Follow these steps exactly!

1. Assess yourself honestly: **start with where you are.** You may be able to start by walking 10 or 15 minutes at a time three or four days a week, or you may be able to start by walking one minute an hour. Either place is fine if it's appropriate for you. **Be realistic about your current level.** If you can walk for 10 minutes, start from that, not by over-optimistically trying to do a half hour right away.

2. State exactly **how much** you will do – that is, how many minutes you will walk. You may decide to follow the suggested progression chart exactly as outlined in Chapter 3, or you may decide to walk for less (or more), depending on your level of readiness.

3. State **when** you will walk. Again, be specific: before breakfast, during your lunch break, immediately after work or an evening walk with the dog.

4. State **how often** you will walk. It usually is best to contract to do something three or four times a week. If you do more, that's a bonus. All people have days when they don't feel like doing anything – so if you say you will walk three or four days a week, you can still meet your contract even if there are days when you don't feel like walking.

5. Once you have made your contract, ask yourself: "On a scale of zero to 10, with zero being totally unsure and 10 being totally certain, **how sure** am I that I can complete this contract?" If your answer is seven or above, you probably have a realistic contract. If your answer is below seven, you should rethink. Ask yourself why are you unsure? What problems do you think you will have? Then figure out if you can solve the problems (for example, using some of the strategies in Chapters 4 and 5). If not, change your contract to be more realistic. This will increase the chances of your success.

6. Determine a **reward** to give yourself for completing your contract. It should be something meaningful to you that you feel would be celebratory of a job well done. Your reward can be anything you decide – from a new pair of walking shoes, to a celebration, like a healthy dinner with your family or friends, to an

evening out dancing. (See the end of this chapter for more on rewards.) Include this reward on your contract.

7. Once you have made a contract you are happy with, **write the final contract down** and **post** this sheet where you will see it every day.

A sample contract is provided in the back of this book. Use this contract form to formalize your walking goals and get motivated to begin!

Step 2: Make a Walking Diary

Research also shows that keeping records of your behavior helps you make and maintain changes. Record keeping can be simple or elaborate – what you should do depends on your personality and what seems to work best for you.

See the sample diary. Leave at least enough space to write down how long or how far you walked (your time duration) and your intensity. You might also want to occasionally record the results of any self-tests (see next section), or make brief notes about your reactions (what you liked, your level of comfort, anything that made exercising difficult on a particular day).

A sample walking diary is included at the end of the book. Use this sample diary or create your own in a bound notebook or journal.

Step 3: Do Some Self-Test Measurements

You don't have to do this step – but it really is a good way to see your progress by giving you a concrete measurement of your starting point at the beginning of your contract. Self-tests aren't complicated – in fact, they're easy.

You can measure the amount of time you are able to walk, or the distance you are able to walk, or take a physical measurement such as your heart rate. If you choose to do this step, see Chapter 6 for a complete description of some recommended self-tests. Record the date and results on your *Walk With Ease* diary. If you don't do this step now, you may later decide that it's a good idea – self-tests are especially valuable if done at the start and end of a contract period, but don't forget they can be done at any point you like!

Step 4: Start Your Program and Record Your Activity

Record at least the time duration of your walk on your diary each day. It's important to keep track of how much you walk so you can keep an eye on your progress. You may also be able to notice trouble spots, such as times when you find it difficult to walk or when you don't have time to walk as far as you normally do.

Step 5: Repeat the Self-Tests at Regular Intervals

If you choose to do self-tests, repeat them every few weeks (a three or four week interval is fine) and record the results on your diary. Chances are, you'll see some progress – for example, you may be able to walk farther than before, or be able to walk comfortably for more minutes at a time.

However, don't be concerned if you note little or no change – it doesn't matter how quickly you progress, just keep it up. It is much more important to gradually make permanent changes than to push for a major change that you are unable to sustain.

Step 6: Check Results/Revise Your Program Every Week

At the end of each week, take stock of your program. For example, are you feeling less fatigued? Are you enjoying yourself? Do you see changes in your self-tests? Also, check on how well you have fulfilled your contract.

If you are having difficulty, this is a good time to use "consultants" to help you accomplish your goal. Depending on the problem (motivation, logistics, pain), your consultants may be friends, family, exercise leaders or health-care providers. Then, as with any plan that may need modifying, make changes if necessary. Decide what worked and what made exercising difficult.

If you have been making notes, look over your diary for ideas. Think about your program. Modify your plan if you need to. You may decide to change the place or time you exercise, your exercise partners, your routes, your pain management strategies or other things that will make your program more enjoyable and successful.

Step 7: Reward Yourself For Accomplishing Your Goals

It's a good idea to give yourself rewards as you go along – not necessarily with expensive treats or with junk food, but by incorporating things that are pleasant and meaningful to you.

For example, if you enjoy watching TV in the evening, you might put it off until after you've walked. The pleasurable act of watching your favorite program turns into a reward for accomplishing your daily goal. You also could give yourself a small treat at the halfway point or at other set intervals during your contract period. Treats could be anything from a walk to the mall, to a new exercise book, to a sunrise walk with a special friend. Think of things that would be pleasurable to you – and plan to give yourself some of these at intervals throughout your contract.

When you complete your contract, give yourself a congratulatory reward for your dedication and success. Of course, the best reward is accomplishing your goal! But also congratulate yourself with that special treat that you decided would be a reward for your completion of your contract – the new pair of walking shoes, the celebratory healthy dinner, for example.

Step 8: Make a New Contract

At the end of your contract period, assess your progress and contract for another few weeks based on your *new (*or continuing) goals.* Simply follow steps 1-7 again!

Self-Check

❑ I have appropriate equipment for walking, including shoes, socks, clothing and any aids I need.

❑ I understand the F.I.T. principles of walking.

❑ I am confident I can complete my walking contract.

Remember

Developing a plan to succeed will improve your chances of success!

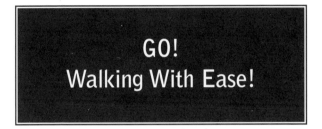

CHAPTER 3

GO!
Walking With Ease!

Now that you know the basics of F.I.T. exercise and have a plan, you are ready to go. This chapter will take you through the practical steps of building your walking program, including lots of good suggestions from exercise experts for ensuring comfort, safety and success.

Implementing the Five-Step Basic Walking Pattern

As you start to implement your plan, here's some basic information to help you get off on the right foot (so to speak). Whenever you go walking for a minimum of 10 minutes, regardless of your ability or speed, follow these steps:

Five-step walking pattern:

1. Start walking at a slow pace to warm up.
2. Gently stretch.
3. Speed up (even a little).
4. Cool down (allow heart rate to recover or return to a more resting level).
5. Stretch gently.

What if you walk for less than 10 minutes at a time? Actually, the five-step general pattern is a good one for you to follow, too. Just start walking slowly, stretch a little, walk a little faster, slowdown and stretch again! These steps are further described below.

Step 1: Walk Slowly To Warm Up (three to five minutes)

Warming up is very important before active exercise, because it prepares you both physically (by warming up muscles and preparing you for exercise, elevating temperature and increasing blood flow) and mentally (by helping you focus and get energized) for the moderate walk to come. To warm up, all you need to do is:

- Stroll or walk at a slow pace for about three to five minutes. (Alternatively, you can march in place or walk around your house for the warm-up time.)

- As you walk or march, roll your shoulders and reach your arms overhead to warm your upper body.

Step 2: Gently Stretch (three to four minutes)

Doing leg and body stretches will help prevent shin pain, sore muscles and other injuries, especially as you go for longer walks. Be sure to do each stretch with both your right and left sides. **Hold each stretch for 20 to 30 seconds and do not bounce.** (See Appendix A for exercise directions and pictures.)

- Upper calf and hip

- Lower calf and Achilles tendon

- Sides and arms

- Other stretches (included in the back of this book)

Step 3: Walk Faster (five to 30 minutes or more)

This is the "aerobic" part of your walk. Follow these guidelines:

- Gradually pick up your pace until you are walking at a moderate pace. Walk as if you have somewhere to go!

- To gradually increase your time, follow the suggested walking progression chart on page 56 as a guideline. If you are a beginner start by walking a total of 10 minutes: a three-to-five minute faster segment surrounded by your warm-up and cool-down strolls. If you already can walk for longer than 10 minutes at a time, enter the chart at your current level of duration and go from there.

- Use the talk test to monitor yourself: you should still be able to carry on a conversation even when walking at a faster pace. If you can't talk without a lot of huffing and puffing or other discomfort, your pace is too fast; slow down to a more comfortable level! Adjust your pace accordingly.

- As you become more fit (able to walk for longer times or at a faster pace or intensity), be sure to keep your heart rate within the moderate intensity level. Monitor yourself at least occasionally by using the perceived exertion scale or heart rate scale you will learn about in Chapter 6. (These scales help you measure how much your body is working as you exercise. Your numbers should remain in the moderate ranges: from 4 to 7 on the perceived exertion scale, or within the 60 percent to 75 percent range for your age level on the heart rate scale.)

- Use good body mechanics (good posture and efficient body movements) when walking. These are noted in the following section. Try to observe all techniques to help ensure safety and prevent discomfort.

- Avoid common walking "errors" such as overstriding (taking steps that are too long for comfort) or leaning. These also are identified in a later section in this chapter. Be sure to follow suggestions to eliminate or correct potential problems.

Step 4: Cool Down (three to five minutes)

At the end of your walk, slow your pace to a stroll until your heart rate has returned to your pre-walk level.

- Please don't skip this, no matter how hurried you might be. A gradual cool down allows your body to "down-shift" from high gear to a lower gear and finally back to the low gear of everyday movement. Cooling down lets your heart rate lower gradually and prevents your blood from pooling in your legs, which can cause light headedness, dizziness or even fainting.

- To cool down, gradually slow your walking pace to a stroll during the last 3 to 5 minutes of your walk. You should be at no more than a fairly light intensity level. (If you measure your intensity, this level would be 3 or less on the perceived exertion scale, or 10 to 14 beats on the 10-second heart rate scale.)

Step 5: Final Stretch (four to five minutes)

This is the most neglected part of a good walking program. Stretching after exercise helps you prevent soreness, increase flexibility and maintain range of motion.

Repeat the same stretches you did during your warm up but hold each stretch for 30 to 45 seconds. Do not bounce and remember to breathe! (See Appendix A for exercise directions and pictures.)

Suggested Walking Progression

When you can walk for a total of 10 minutes at a time (including warm up and cool down), follow this suggested walking progression chart to gradually build your fitness program. If you already can walk for longer than 10 minutes at a time, enter the chart at your current level and progress accordingly.

Week	Time Duration Per Walking Session*	Frequency Per Week
1	10 minutes	3-5 times
2	15 minutes	3-5 times
3	20 minutes	3-5 times
4	25 minutes	3-5 times
5	30 minutes	3-5 times
6	30-35 minutes	3-5 times
7	30-40 minutes	3-5 times
8	30-45 minutes	3-5 times
9	30-50 minutes	3-5 times

10 and onward Keep your walks at 30-60 minutes per session, 3-5 times a week. Gradually increase your intensity until you are in the moderate range (if you are not doing so yet).

*includes warm-up and cool-down strolls, but not stretching

Remember, this program as described is a suggested goal. You may not be able to walk this long right away or progress as quickly as outlined. Or you may "top out" and be unable to add time duration beyond a certain point. That's OK. It is important to start at your current level, build up gradually and slowly increase your time to your maximum ability in order to increase your stamina and muscle strength.

Comfort, Safety and Other Tips

1. If you feel any of the following symptoms, STOP immediately – these are danger signs. If these persist, get medical help or call 911:

- Severe pain

- Pressure, tightness or pain in your chest

- Nausea

- Difficulty with breathing

- Dizziness

- Severe trembling

- Light-headedness

2. If you have any of the following symptoms, SLOW DOWN immediately – these are signs you are overexerting yourself. Cut back on your walking intensity or duration the next time you exercise:

- Cramps or stitches in your side

- Very red face

- Sudden paling or blanching

- Profuse sweating

- Facial expression signifying distress

- Extreme tiredness

- Fatigue or joint pain that lasts two hours after exercising (and is greater than you had before you started)

3. These reactions to exercise are normal; it's OK to continue

- Increased breathing

- Increased heart rate

- Increased perspiration

- Muscle soreness

Note: Some muscle soreness often develops a day or two after you exercise, particularly if you are just beginning your program. Take warm baths, stretch gently and continue to walk. However, use common sense. If you have severe pain, see numbers 1 and 2 above.

4. Always empty your bladder before exercising. (Note: if you frequently have to go to the bathroom or experience the common dilemma of "leaking," see suggestions in Chapter 4.)

5. Using heat or cold before exercise may help relax muscles and joints and get you ready to go. Other pain-management strategies also may be helpful. (See suggestions in Chapter 5.)

6. Light self-massage before your warm up may be helpful if muscles or joints are stiff. However, do not massage painful joints.

7. Most people should drink plenty of fluids after each workout, whether you feel thirsty or not. Water is essential to satisfy your body's need for fluid, especially when you perspire. If it's very hot or you know you're going to be walking for a long time, you might want to take along a water bottle in a fanny pack or backpack. (Note: Be especially aware of drinking enough water when you walk in humid weather, since you are less conscious of fluid loss.)

8. It is perfectly safe to exercise while menstruating. In fact, many women find that exercise helps reduce cramps or other uncomfortable menstrual symptoms.

9. If you are unable to walk during one of your planned times because of weather or emergencies, that's OK – but immediately decide when you will schedule in the next session.

10. Remember that symptoms of arthritis come and go. Exercise that seems easy one day may seem too hard the next. When this happens, cut back temporarily and then return to your regular program when you can.

Good Body Mechanics

Good body mechanics are efficient movements that produce the least stress on your body and reduce the likelihood of injuries or problems:

- Swing your arms naturally and easily at your sides, with your arms moving opposite to your legs (i.e., your right arm swings forward as you step with your left leg, then your left arm swings forward as you step with your right leg).

- Keep your head up, chin neutral. Don't jut your head forward or lead with your chin.

- Stand tall and elongate your chest. You should lift your rib cage and you should not slump your chest and shoulders.

- Tighten your stomach muscles lightly to maintain good back support.

- Periodically think about your shoulders to be sure they are relaxed and down (not hunched). If you are hunching, lift your rib cage up and do a few backward shoulder circles to relax your shoulders.

- Breathe deeply from your lungs and diaphragm. Avoid shallow breathing with only your upper lungs.

- Don't clench your fists – just hold your hands naturally. If you have a tendency to clench, imagine you have fragile raw eggs in your hands as you swing your arms naturally.

- Be careful not to overstride, which wastes energy and increases impact. Especially avoid the natural tendency to take longer strides as you become more fit, or when it's a beautiful day and you just feel great! Take regular, natural steps that are comfortable with your tempo. If you need to reduce impact, take even shorter steps.

Strengthening and Range-of-Motion Exercises

If you have a form of arthritis that involves the knees, ankles or hips, you should do the following exercises to help strengthen the supporting muscles and to help you walk more comfortably. If you have ongoing, severe pain in your knees, ankles or hips, you should talk to your doctor or physical therapist to get specific exercise recommendations. (See exercise directions and illustrations in Appendix A.)

Knees
1. Quadriceps lifts
2. Ready to go

Hips and Legs
1. Down and ups

Ankles and Feet
1. Ankle rotations
2. Foot raise

Remember that this book focuses on the development of a walking program and does not contain information about other kinds of strengthening and flexibility exercises you should be doing as part of your arthritis management program. Consult other references (see Chapter 7) or talk to your doctor or physical therapist for suggestions.

Common Problems and Solutions
Sore Shins (Shin Splints)

Sore shins can stem from several causes. One common cause is inadequate warming up and stretching. Another is doing too much, too fast. A third could be shoes that are too big, too old or provide poor support.

To prevent sore shins, always start with good shoes that are properly fitted. Keep your feet and toes relaxed while you're walking, and avoid gripping shoes with your toes. (If you find yourself "gripping," that's a sign that your shoes are probably too big.) Always start walking with a strolling warm up and stretch, and always cool down gradually and stretch again. Be especially careful to build your walking duration slowly. Do ankle flexibility exercises and stretch your shins daily. One move you can try is the ankle rotation exercise in Appendix A.

Sore Knees

You may be walking too fast or on a surface level that's too stressful. Slow down a little and keep your stride short. To slow your speed but keep your heart rate up, try doing more work with your arms, if you comfortably can. This may include a good arm swinging motion – see "elbow whipping" below for more guidance in this area. Be sure you are reducing impact as much as possible (review the section "A Note About Impact" in Chapter 2). Additionally do leg-strengthening exercises to help reduce overall knee pain (see the quadriceps lift, ready to go, and down and ups exercises in Appendix A). Shoe problems can show up in your knees as well as your feet, so make sure your shoes provide good support and cushioning (review "Shoes" in Chapter 2).

Calf Cramps

Often the culprit for calf cramps is lack of adequate stretching before and after walking, so be sure you warm up and stretch properly. Dehydration also can cause leg cramps; be careful to drink lots of fluids while exercising.

If you have circulatory problems in the legs and experience cramping while walking, alternate intervals of brisk and slow walking. If persistent, check with your doctor or physical therapist. To help prevent cramps, wear shoes that fit properly and provide adequate support and cushioning (again, review "Shoes" in Chapter 2).

Heel Pain

Again, inadequate stretching before and after walking is often the reason for heel pain. Be sure to warm up and stretch properly. Shoes that provide adequate support and cushioning, particularly in the heel will also help. If, despite taking these precautions, your heel pain persists, check with your doctor or therapist to be sure your plantar fascia has not become inflamed. He or she may also be able to suggest particular stretches to help you avoid heel pain.

Overstriding

If your hair or hat bounces up and down when you walk, it's a good indication you are overstriding. Sometimes when you feel great and you're enjoying yourself, you may have a natural tendency to do this – but remember, it increases impact and adds stress to your hips, knees and feet. Try to glide along the ground and take shorter, more natural steps.

Elbow Whipping

A good arm swing comes naturally from the shoulder, not up and down from the elbow. While it's fine to keep your elbows in a comfortable, natural bend, avoid "whipping" the forearms up and down from a bent elbow. Avoid a "rocking the baby" motion if you can.

Waist Leaning

An ache in your lower back after walking often is the result of tilting forward and letting your buttocks stick out. Try to maintain neutral posture and avoid a forward lean.

To feel the difference, stand with your back against a wall and then lean slightly forward while leaving your buttocks against the wall – that's not the position you want to be in when walking! Now stand with your back against the wall and lean slightly forward from your ankles – that's the proper forward lean.

Slumping

Slumping puts pressure on your back and causes a number of other problems. Review the previous section on good body mechanics – keep your chest up, abdominal muscles in and shoulders relaxed and down.

Self-Check

❏ I understand the importance of all five phases of walking: the warm up, the stretch, the faster walk, the cool down and the final stretch.

❏ I can observe good walking principles and body mechanics.

❏ I am confident I can implement my walking program successfully!

Remember

Enjoy the good feelings and all the benefits that regular walking brings to you. Just a little extra effort each day means a lifetime of better health.

CHAPTER 4

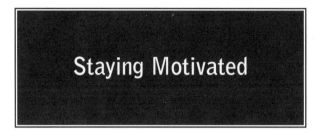

Staying Motivated

Do you remember the six stages of change described
in the introduction? Many people who start exercising
end up dropping out before they get to Stage 5 (the stage
of successful maintenance) because they run into obstacles that affect their motivation. Motivation is not some
mysterious quality that some people have and others are
lacking – the real way to achieve success is to find ways
to help overcome problems that loom in your way.

Develop Strategies To Overcome Difficulties

Everyone runs into problems in developing and sticking
with an exercise program. Here are some of the solutions
used by successful exercisers with arthritis to counteract
obstacles and stay motivated. See if they can help you, too.

Possible Solutions:

I Have Medical Problems.

A. Even with medical problems, chances are that you can do appropriate exercises. Talk with your doctor, physical therapist or fitness professional to answer your specific questions and help develop a safe, effective program. Take this book along and use it as a basis to discuss what is right for you. Remember, nearly everyone with medical problems can and should exercise.

B. If you have certain severe medical conditions or symptoms, you should consult your doctor before undertaking any form of exercise. If you have any of the conditions listed in Chapter 1, you may need to exercise in a supervised program; that is, with a trained medical staff person.

C. If you are having an arthritis flare, don't skip your exercises entirely. Get plenty of rest, but maintain gentle range-of-motion exercises. As the flare settles down, begin some strengthening exercises. Get back to your walking program as soon as you can. Review Chapter 1 for additional information about the harm too much rest can cause and the importance of balancing rest and activity.

I Have Tried Before, but It Hurt and I Had To Stop.

A. You may have tried to do too much or do it too fast. Carefully review the guidelines in our program so you can progress in a safe and effective manner without soreness, muscle strains, excess joint discomfort or injury. Also, make sure you are exercising appropriately for your ability and specific form of arthritis. Review Chapter 1 and talk to your doctor or therapist if you need advice.

B. Was it joint pain? If so, heat or cold often can be helpful. Try using heat before exercise (heating pads, hot showers, warm tub baths) to help warm up joints, reduce stiffness and relax muscles. Use cold after exercise (ice, cold packs or even bags of frozen vegetables) on any sore joints. Never use heat or cold for more than 20 minutes. See Chapter 5 for additional heat and cold suggestions.

C. Maybe you need to try a different form of exercise that puts less strain on your body. Walking is a good exercise for most people, but if walking continues to be a problem, try aquatic exercise as your aerobic activity, since it minimizes joint discomfort.

D. For many people with arthritis, exercise may cause some temporary joint discomfort. But rest assured, proper exercise will not further damage or injure joints and in fact helps. Use the two-hour pain rule described in Chapter 1, and exercise appropriately for your ability level. Don't use the "no pain, no gain" mentality – pain does not indicate that you are "working out" at a more effective level. Some soreness may occur when you are first getting into activity, but if you experience pain that is long-lasting or intense, you need to consult your doctor or physical therapist.

I Don't Have Time.

A. If you work for eight to nine hours a day and sleep for another eight or nine, that leaves six to eight hours every day for other activities – including weekends, you have 60 to 72 hours each week. Just two hours of that time is all you need for a great investment for your health!

B. Think of walking as a special time when you are focused on taking care of yourself. Even for just a few minutes a day, you're actively improving your health, relieving stress and taking care of your body. Use this time to think about other creative goals for yourself.

C. Actually, few of us have the time to exercise. We have to make the time. One good way is to make appointments with yourself by writing your walking times in your daily calendar just like you do business meetings, doctors' appointments or other important things.

D. Combine your walk with another activity. Have a "walking meeting" with a friend or business colleague. Or catch up on the news with friends or neighbors while you walk, instead of using the phone. Or if you can use a treadmill comfortably, put one in front of the TV and walk while you watch the news or your favorite show. Try walking a pet, such as an active dog. Encourage your spouse or family members to join you in a group walk.

E. Many people find that scheduling walks for the same time on every exercise day helps them make walking a routine part of their schedule. Whether it's early in the morning, during your lunch break, after work or later in the evening, figure out a time that works best for you. Put your scheduled walk on your to-do list or calendar just as you record your business meetings and social obligations.

F. Look for activities you do now that you might be willing to give up to make time to help yourself be more fit and healthier. It might be a few minutes of TV time, reading, meeting time or time talking on the phone. Maybe you can "give up" something you don't even like!

I'm Too Tired.

A. There are several causes for fatigue: 1) physical (lack of sleep, muscle weakness, poor nutrition, physical exertion, side effects of certain medicine), 2) emotional (stress, depression, effort of coping) or 3) a combination. Try to figure out why you are tired and address these areas if possible – for example, get more good-quality sleep, lose some weight, strengthen muscles, practice relaxation techniques or eat a proper diet. Correcting these kinds of underlying problems will help you feel better and have much more energy.

B. One of the major causes of fatigue actually can be lack of exercise. Therefore, exercise like walking can help you be less tired. Even if you feel fatigued, try just a little exercise – say, a five-minute walk. You may be surprised!

C. When you think you're really too tired, force yourself to walk for just two minutes. If you are still too tired to exercise, then stop. Many times you'll feel energized enough to keep going!

D. It's a funny thing, but regular exercise really does make you more energetic. Besides making you stronger, exercise stimulates your body to pump out endorphins (the feel-good hormones) and reduces stress – both of which make you feel better and more "up and at 'em." Think of what you're not getting when you're not walking regularly.

E. OK, if you really are fatigued, rest for a while. Then walk!

I Just Don't Feel Like it.

A. Find an exercise partner. Schedule regular times for walks so you will need to be there for your fitness buddy.

B. Join a group of people who need someone to walk with. Look for a walking group at your community center, church, Arthritis Foundation chapter, Parks and Recreation Department or YMCA/YWCA. If there isn't one, you can start one of your own: just round up an informal group of your friends or neighbors and schedule regular times to meet for walks. (Call the Arthritis Foundation if you'd like more information about joining or starting a *Walk With Ease* group.) Groups are a great way to keep each other going during times when it's easier not to go.

C. Consider getting a dog. Seriously! Having to take an animal for a walk ensures that you do, too. (Additionally, studies show that dog-owners have lower stress levels and live longer.) For walking purposes, be sure to choose a breed that is appropriate for your own ability – talk to a vet or animal trainer for recommendations.

D. Picture in your mind what you really want for yourself out of exercise. More energy? Less joint pain? Fitter body? Stronger bones? Focus on that vision, rather than on the thought that you don't feel like exercising right now.

E. It may surprise you that even long-time, avid exercisers often don't feel like exercising either. But they know they will feel good afterwards. They focus on long-term achievements instead of short-term gratification.

The Weather is Bad.

A. Go to the mall! Lots of people, especially in bad weather, go mall-walking. If a mall isn't convenient, how about a supermarket, an airport concourse, a community center or an indoor track? Anywhere under cover works. In fact, some malls and community areas already have regularly scheduled walks during early or late hours for people just like you.

B. It never rains or snows on a treadmill. Good, inexpensive treadmills can be purchased to substitute for outdoor walking when the weather is just too nasty to go outside. (Note that a treadmill may not be a good choice if you have balance problems or difficulty with your hands.) Consult *Consumer Reports* in your library or online, or call your YMCA for recommendations.

C. Focus on your strengthening and stretching exercises when the weather is too bad to go outside. Staying active doing household chores and dancing to your favorite music will help you maintain the aerobic fitness you have achieved through your walking program.

I Don't Feel Safe When I Walk.

A. Walk during times of day when light and shadows don't cause problems with your vision. If there's little light during your walking time, wear bright, reflective clothing or reflectors so drivers can see you. Carry a flashlight after dusk.

B. Avoid areas where there might be a threat to your personal safety. Use community walking areas such as schools, parks, indoor tracks or recreation centers.

C. Be sure a family member or friend knows your walking route and approximately how long you'll be gone.

D. Remember that a walking stick not only helps with balance and joint comfort, it also is a handy defense against dogs or other aggressors. In fact, many people both with and without arthritis regularly walk with sticks for that very purpose.

E. Walk with a buddy or group. Ask your neighbors if they would like to start walking with you. There's safety in numbers, plus it's a good way to prevent boredom.

F. It's OK to stay close to home. You can walk a mile by going up and down the same block five to seven times.

G. If you're concerned about getting too tired before you get home, consider buying a walking stick with a collapsing seat so you can rest whenever you need to.

I Need To Use the Bathroom Frequently.

A. Lots of people experience this problem. If necessary, stay close to home or in areas where you know you can find a bathroom when you need one.

B. Plan walking routes in advance, noting bathroom availability so you're less likely to be caught by surprise.

C. Always remember to empty your bladder before you start to walk.

D. Wear appropriate pads or protective undergarments. Don't let this problem become a barrier to your fitness.

My Feet Hurt When I Walk.

A. Make sure your shoes provide good support, are fitted properly, are the right kind of shoe for your activity and are not old or worn out. (Review shoe guidelines in Chapter 2.)

B. Do you have bunions, corns, plantar fasciitis, arch problems or another foot condition that causes discomfort (other than arthritis)? If so, see your doctor for a course of treatment. Also, since many of these problems are caused or made worse by poor-fitting or certain styles of shoes, be sure all your shoes fit your feet properly. Chances are, these problems can be treated or corrected – don't let them affect the rest of your health.

C. Maintain a healthy weight. Every extra pound on your body puts three to four extra pounds of pressure on your feet (and also on your knees, hips and back), so maintaining a healthy weight is important for your feet and joints. (Regular walking helps you maintain a good weight!)

D. Be sure your walking technique is good. Review good body mechanics in Chapter 3, and note especially the paragraphs concerning sore feet and knees.

E. You might consider adding an extra layer of cushioning in your shoes by inserting insoles that you can buy at a drugstore or shoe store. Remember that insoles (the ones that come in shoes when you buy them) usually wear out faster than the shoes themselves, so you should replace insoles every few months to maintain good cushioning.

NOTE: Some people may need to have special orthotic inserts in their shoes. If your feet continue to hurt, discuss this option with your doctor.

I'm Stiff/Unsteady on My Feet. I Don't Like To Be Seen Staggering. People Will Think I'm Drunk.

A. If you have never used a walking stick, it might be enough to provide the support you need. Go at your own pace, using your stick for balance.

B. Many of the problems that are attributed to arthritis, such as stiffness and hesitant gait, often are the result of inactivity, not arthritis itself. For many people, getting up and going is the key to less stiffness, better body mechanics, and to feeling and doing better on their feet.

C. Who cares about what inconsiderate or judgmental people think? Actually, most of us do care what others think – and we can help educate thoughtless people by being good role models. For example, call attention to your efforts by wearing an Arthritis Foundation T-shirt or one with a special exercise phrase. Seeing people with arthritis who are successfully exercising despite limitations can help others think twice about their assumptions – and you'll be a great example and get your exercise.

D. If you're still uncomfortable about this, walk with a group or in an area where you *are* comfortable.

I Think Exercise Clothing Looks Ridiculous.

A. If you don't want to wear special exercise-type clothes, you don't have to. Wear a T-shirt or sweatshirt, shorts or pants – or whatever you want to wear. That's the beauty of walking. All you really need are good shoes and socks and the right clothing for the weather.

B. Some people who try fitness clothing find it to be very comfortable. Walking shorts and other special exercise clothing are made of fabrics that provide good support and help regulate temperature. You might actually like it!

I Don't Like To Sweat.

A. Sweating is your body's natural air-conditioning system. If you sweat during exercise, it's usually a good sign – it means you are exerting yourself enough to generate energy, burn calories and make changes that benefit your health.

B. For comfort, you can wear clothing that helps absorb or wick perspiration from your body so you don't feel as uncomfortable when you sweat. Review Chapter 2 for some suggestions.

C. Actually, you don't have to sweat a lot to get the benefits of exercise. Remember the FIT principles discussed in Chapter 2. Low intensity activity is fine – just do it for a little longer time duration. (Although we hope you'll be enjoying yourself so much that it doesn't matter whether or not you sweat!)

I'm Too Old and/or Out of Shape To Exercise.

A. It is never too late to start exercising! It doesn't matter how old or out of shape you are now – your body will receive the same benefits from walking that younger or more active people receive.

B. Almost all the things that get worse with age get better with exercise – so while it's good to exercise when you're younger, it is essential to exercise as you get older. Even if you have never been active before, you will receive benefits to your health as soon as you start exercising.

C. If you're older or out of shape, you may need to go a little slower than you might have a few years ago, but that's perfectly OK. Go at whatever speed and comfort you need – the important thing is to get going.

I Had To Miss a Few Times and It's Hard To Get Started Again.

A. A lapse is just that – a lapse. Don't let it become a collapse! Even long-time, dedicated exercisers have occasional lapses. If you miss doing your walks for a short period of time, interpret that as just a lapse – and make a firm decision to get right back on the exercise track.

B. Remember, there actually are predictable dropout periods that all exercisers struggle through. Realize these are coming, and plan to get through times when it's hard to get going by doing some of the other strategies mentioned in this section. Missing a few times is perfectly OK – just get right back with your program to avoid becoming a permanent exercise dropout.

My Doctor Has:

Not Told Me I Should Walk.

A. Have you ever discussed walking with your doctor? Often, it never comes up! During busy office visits many doctors don't think to mention something as simple as walking. If your arthritis is not particularly complicated, walking probably isn't a problem at all – try following the guidelines and see how you feel.

B. If you have concerns, take this book to your doctor and be prepared with specific questions to ask concerning exercise guidelines for you. Be sure to refer to overall exercise guidelines in Chapter 1, sections on time duration and intensity in Chapter 2, and the five-step walking pattern in Chapter 3. Chances are you'll be able to start a program. If your doctor does say you shouldn't walk, discuss alternative ways in which you can get needed exercise.

Said I Should Be Careful Not To Overdo it When I Exercise.

A. That's excellent advice for everyone. Follow the guidelines in our program – especially review Chapters 1-3. Start with what you can do, progress very slowly and gradually, and make any modifications you need for your form of arthritis or related condition. Take this book to your doctor and discuss what you should do.

Exercise Is Boring.

A. Keep variety in your exercise routine. For example, walk different routes – try different streets in the neighborhood or totally different areas. Walk with different friends on various days of the week. Listen to music or books on tape on your headphones (but be careful for safety – don't lose connection with your surroundings and don't lose focus on your balance). There are hundreds of ways to make walking more fun.

B. Find exercises that you like to do. If you don't like walking, try a low-impact aerobics class, tai chi, swimming, bicycling or whatever. Keep trying until you find something you think is enjoyable. You will!

C. Distract yourself by walking with a buddy (as mentioned above) or family members. Schedule walks with your partner, children or grandchildren for quality time and good health together.

D. Set different goals for yourself. Focus one day on improving your time, another day on alternating speeds, another day on stopping to smell the flowers (or whatever else you might enjoy). Every once in a while, enjoy a nice, leisurely stroll as a treat.

E. As a last resort, just reconcile yourself to being bored for a while! (This might be necessary especially if you have to walk in the same area all the time, such as around a track.) Try all the other techniques to reduce boredom, but if worse comes to worse, remember: You probably do other things that are a little boring or that you don't really like either, but you do them because the benefits outweigh your feelings. Think of exercise in the same way – and just do it.

I Am Afraid Walking Will Make My Arthritis Worse.

A. As mentioned before, if you are concerned about walking, take this book along with you to your doctor and discuss appropriate exercise for you.

B. A significant number of research studies now prove that appropriate exercise will not make arthritis and related conditions worse and, in fact, will help decrease overall pain and make you feel better. This is true for almost all people with arthritis: You will not hurt yourself with appropriate exercise, but you will hurt yourself by not exercising! If your condition is not particularly limiting, you can start on your own and follow our recommended guidelines. If you do have limitations, talk with your doctor before starting anything. It is likely that regular exercise like walking will help you manage your condition and feel better.

Exercise Is Not a Priority for Me Compared to Other Things I Need To Do.

Possible solutions:

A. You may have many obligations in your life: family, spouse, work, volunteer work, household maintenance, religion, etc. But your health should be a major priority. A key component of staying healthy is regular exercise – particularly if you have arthritis.

B. Exercising regularly will give you the energy you need to complete all the tasks on your to-do list. If you have arthritis, and you don't stay active, your pain and stiffness will grow worse. Exercise will reduce your pain and stiffness, help you sleep better and boost your energy level to enable you to do what you have to do now and more.

Develop and Maintain Support

You have a greater chance of successfully keeping up your walking plan if your family, friends and co-workers are supportive, rather than being indifferent to your efforts. You can generate your own cheering squad by doing some specific planning. Here are a few suggestions:

Spouse or Partner

Your spouse or partner is probably one of the most important people in your life. He or she can have a major impact in your attempts to maintain motivation.

Ask your partner to join you on some of your walks. Discuss daily events, family issues or the news. Both of you will reap the benefits of walking – and you may even find a bonus in your relationship!

Family Members

Do you have children or grandchildren? Take them for a walk, to the park or the zoo, or on some other outing that requires walking. Besides getting your own walk, you'll be serving as a good example that physical activity is fun and important. And remember, adult children like these things, too.

Friends and Co-Workers

Find exercise buddies. Arrange for a morning walk with a friend. It's not as easy to roll over and go back to sleep if you know your exercise partner is waiting. Meet a co-worker at lunchtime and walk together to a cafeteria or restaurant nearby.

Exercise Role Models

No, not star athletes or famous movie stars, but real people you admire for their exercise habits. Maybe a friend who has severe arthritis but who walks regularly. Maybe a particularly motivated person in your walking group. Talk to these people about how and why they keep to their walking program. If they can do it, so can you.

Walking Group

If you don't belong to one already, think about joining a *Walk With Ease* group. If there isn't one in your area, think about starting one! Contact your local chapter of the Arthritis Foundation for more information. At the end of this book, we'll show you how to find your local chapter and the many resources available there.

Self-Check

❑ I have a plan to overcome barriers that interfere with walking.

❑ I feel confident that I have the tools to get past setbacks and obstacles.

❑ I can develop a support system that helps me keep going.

Remember

Setbacks are normal. Don't let small lapses become a collapse!

CHAPTER 5

Making a Plan To Manage Pain

Understanding Pain

Most people with arthritis have pain. For many, it is the number one concern, and all too often it becomes a barrier to successfully sticking to an exercise program.

Remember, the pain caused by arthritis and related conditions comes from at least three sources:

- **Damaged and/or inflamed joints and other tissues.** This is the pain caused directly by the condition.

- **Weak, tense muscles.** When a joint is damaged, the natural response of the body is to protect the joint by tensing surrounding muscles. Unfortunately, many people have weak muscles that can't take the stress. Additionally, tense muscles themselves cause pain by building up lactic acid. Try holding your arm straight out to your side for five minutes to verify the discomfort that comes from muscle tension.

- **Fear and depression.** When you are upset or depressed everything seems worse, including pain.

Regular physical activity plays a big role in managing overall pain by helping protect joints, making supporting muscles stronger, reducing muscular stress, lessening depression and helping you just feel better.

But, as we have pointed out many times, exercise itself may include some accompanying discomfort. If you have some pain during or immediately after walking, remember that hurt doesn't necessarily equal harm. For almost everyone, walking does not cause further damage to your joints. It does bring many health and wellness benefits.

To prevent or reduce the discomfort that may accompany exercise, use recommended pain-management techniques as you continue your *Walk With Ease* program.

Tips For Managing Pain

You don't want to let pain keep you from getting beneficial exercise or from doing other things you want to do. While there will be some days that your pain keeps you from certain activities, there are many ways you can help control your pain.

Here are some simple tips to help you manage pain and discomfort so you can keep walking. Once you have found several you like or find helpful, think how you will use each one. Then, place some clues in your environment to remind yourself about your pain-management techniques. For example, place some reminder stickers or notes where you will see them – on your bathroom mirror, the dashboard of your car, your computer monitor, your gym bag. Or have a friend or family member remind you. These kinds of things may seem simple or silly, but research proves they help.

Maintain an Appropriate Weight

If you are overweight, consider losing excess pounds.

- Why? Every extra pound on your body puts several extra pounds of pressure on your hips, knees, ankles and feet. It also stresses your back. Although it's a long-term solution, maintaining a healthy weight usually is one of the best things anyone can do to help prevent or minimize discomfort in your back, hips and lower extremities.

- Remember, walking and weight control go hand and hand. Developing a regular walking program can help you maintain your weight, which will help you walk more comfortably!

Use Medicines for Relief as Advised by Your Doctor

Be sure to check with your doctor before taking anything, even over-the-counter drugs, to be certain the medicine or dosage is appropriate for you.

- Acetaminophen (*Tylenol*) often helps relieve minor pain or discomfort.

- NSAIDS (non-steroidal anti-inflammatory drugs) such as aspirin (*Anacin*), ibuprofen (*Advil* or *Motrin*), and naproxen sodium (*Aleve*) reduce both pain and inflammation. If you get an upset stomach that doesn't go away, call your doctor.

- If you take medicines, plan your walk for when the medicine has maximal effect. That is, give the medicine an hour or two to get into your system.

Follow the Two-Hour Pain Rule

- Remember this rule mentioned throughout the book? If your walking causes pain that continues two hours after walking (which is worse than the pain you had before you started walking), next time slow down and/or decrease the amount of time or the distance you walked. If doing this several times does not help, talk to your health-care provider.

- If you simply are unable to walk more than a very short distance without significant pain, get advice from your doctor or therapist about a different form of exercise that is more appropriate for you.

Use Heat and/or Cold

- Both heat and cold are used for pain relief. Many people find heat most helpful before exercise and cold most helpful after exercise – however, this is up to you. Try for yourself, and use either or both as needed. Heating an inflamed joint is ill-advised, however, because the increased blood flow can make the inflammation worse.

- Heat produces an increase in blood flow, helps reduce stiffness, has a sedative effect on painful nerve endings and relaxes aching muscles and joints. Heating pads, warm showers, warm tub baths or whirlpools (98°F to 102°F) are good sources of heat. Heat treatments should feel soothing and comfortable, not hot.

- Cold applications also can be effective against pain. Cold can help control inflammation and swelling, relieve pain and reduce muscle spasm. Use ice, cold packs or even packages of frozen vegetables wrapped in a towel. (Mark the vegetable bag clearly so you don't eat the contents later!) Some people put popcorn kernels into a plastic bag that, when frozen, works well to mold around a joint.

- Use heat for no more than 20 minutes and cold for no more than 10 to 15 minutes at a time, letting skin return to normal temperature between applications. Also, always remember to protect your skin when using either, by putting a towel or pad between your skin and a heating pad or ice pack.

- Never fall asleep while lying on a heating pad or using an ice pack.

HEAT AND COLD:
Ideas and Tips for Safe, Effective Use

When you experience minor muscle or joint pain, heat and cold treatments can be affordable, effective and easy-to-use solutions. While both heat and cold treatments can be soothing, using them improperly can lead to serious burns or other damaging problems. Use these guidelines and safety tips to make sure you don't hurt yourself while using heat or cold.

- Use heat treatments, such as heating pads, warm towels or warm baths, for soothing stiff joints and tired muscles. Heat helps to make your body limber and ready for exercise or activity.

- Use cold treatments, such as an ice pack, a bag of frozen peas or a cold, wet towel, for acute pain. Cold helps numb the painful spot and decreases inflammation and swelling.

There are many ways to apply heat or cold to your painful areas. Some may work better for you than others. Experiment with these ideas to find out which ones work best for you.

Heat
- Take a long, very warm shower when you first wake up to ease morning stiffness, or before you exercise.

- Use a warm paraffin wax treatment system, available at many drugstores or beauty supply stores. These treatments are effective for use on hands, elbow, feet and ankles.

- Soak in a warm bath, Jacuzzi or whirlpool.

- Buy a moist heat pad from the drugstore. Make your

own by putting a wet washcloth in a freezer bag and heating it in the microwave for 1 minute. Wrap the hot pack in a towel and place it over the affected area for 15 to 20 minutes.

- Incorporate other warming elements into your daily routines, such as warming your clothes in the dryer before dressing or using an electric blanket and turning it up for a few minutes before getting out of bed.

Cold

- Apply a bag of ice wrapped in a towel or gel-filled cold pack from the drugstore to painful areas for about 10 minutes.

- Wrap a towel around a bag of frozen vegetables, such as peas or corn, and place it on painful joints. This type of cold pack easily conforms to your body.

Safety Tips

Follow these guidelines to avoid injury, such as burns or ice burns, when using heat or cold:

- Use the heat or cold therapy for no more than 15 to 20 minutes at a time. Let your skin return to normal temperature before another application.

- Don't place the ice or hot pack directly on your skin — always use a towel in between.

- Never use pain relieving creams or gels with heat treatments.

- Don't sleep with an electric heating pad on.

Apply Gentle, Self-Massage.

- Try lightly massaging stiff or sore areas before exercise. Self-massage stimulates the skin, underlying tissues and muscles by means of applied pressure and stretching. Slow, circular movements or light kneading motions work well for many people. Don't massage one spot for more than 10 to 15 seconds.

- Never massage a joint that is inflamed (hot, red and swollen).

Discuss Using Elastic Supports or Braces With Your Doctor or Physical Therapist.

- Elastic supports can be purchased at drug stores or medical supply stores. If your arthritis is not complicated, these devices can be used to provide some additional walking support for knees or ankles. Discuss with your physical therapist if you are not sure.

- For some people, braces can provide needed knee or ankle support during exercise (just like the support braces some athletes use to protect their knees or ankles during sports activities). And be sure to wear the braces if your doctor suggests them.

Use a Walking Stick or Cane.

These aids can help provide stability and support as you walk, especially if you have hip or knee pain.

- Be sure your stick or cane is the right length. The handle or grip should reach your wrist when your hand is relaxed at your side.

- Check for safety. Walking sticks should be sturdy and have a broad tip. Because the tips of most canes are too small, make your cane more stable by buying a wide rubber tip at any pharmacy.

- Use it correctly – a walking stick or cane should be used on the side opposite your bad side.

Focus on Something Else Other Than Your Pain.

- To take your mind off minor discomfort when walking, think of a person's name, an animal species, an occupation, a movie title or other items in a category for every letter of the alphabet. If you get stuck on one letter (such as X), go on to the next one. Think of a favorite song you haven't sung for a while and try to remember the lyrics. Try naming all the teams in the National Football League or the Atlantic Coast Conference (or whatever you like). Plan walks with a friend so that you can carry on a distracting conversation. There are lots of variations of distraction, once you have the idea.

- However, use common sense. Do not distract yourself when you need to be observant! Distraction is not recommended if you need to concentrate on your balance, your walking technique or your surroundings.

Reinterpret Your Sensations.

- Rather than distracting yourself, think specifically about your physical sensations, but try to interpret them differently. For example, don't think of your symptoms as "pain" or "hurt" (terms that connote danger or distress); instead analyze the precise physical sensations and describe them – hot, sharp or aching?

- See if you can begin to relabel your symptoms as specific kinds of temporary discomfort, not as pain. With practice, this can help you lessen the intensity of your symptoms by training your mind to change the way it thinks about your symptoms. For example, when you first start walking, re-label the stiffness or soreness you feel as a part of getting started. Remind yourself that once you get warmed up, your joints will loosen and feel better. This is hard to do in the beginning, but it will get easier for you if you practice at times other than when walking.

Change Your Self-Talk

- All of us talk to ourselves all the time. Our self-talk comes in many forms, mostly negative, such as "I can't do..." or "If only I didn't...." Research shows that, in particular, this kind of negative self-talk can worsen pain, depression and fatigue. Try to change this.

- To make self-talk work for you instead of against you, try to listen to and analyze your internal thoughts. To start, ask yourself, "What is the evidence to support this? Is my interpretation really correct? What would I say to a friend who was in my shoes?" By asking yourself these simple questions, you may be able to identify more positive and hopeful thoughts about your situation.

Note: The following examples of unrealistic, negative self-talk are common for people with arthritis. If you have similar thoughts, make a conscious effort to replace them with more realistic or balanced thoughts.

Negative self-talk	Balanced self-talk
This pain is terrible.	I've dealt with this problem before.
I can't stand it.	It will get better.
The pain is awful. It's hopeless.	I can do things to control my pain.
It's impossible to walk when I'm in pain.	I hurt, but exercise will strengthen my body.

Self-Check

❏ I can use several of the management strategies to manage my discomfort.

❏ I have planned when I can use these tactics during my walking program, if necessary.

❏ I have placed stickers or notes to remind myself to use these techniques.

Remember

Hurt does not equal harm. Use pain-management strategies to minimize hurt as much as possible.

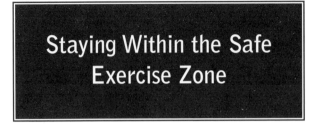

CHAPTER 6

Staying Within the Safe Exercise Zone

Everyone – regardless of age, level of ability or experience – should follow recommended guidelines for safety and comfort when exercising. Many safety recommendations already have been covered throughout the five previous chapters of this book. Here are some additional guidelines to help you maintain safety and keep yourself injury-free.

Monitoring Your Exercise Intensity

Monitoring intensity when you exercise is good for two reasons: 1) It lets you know if you are working hard enough or too hard so that you exercise at a safe and effective level; and 2) It helps provide you with a measuring stick to gauge your progress over time.

There are several good and easy ways to measure your intensity. Try the following techniques.

The Talk Test

This is a quick, informal way to make sure you aren't overdoing it. Simply talk out loud to another person or yourself, sing or recite the verse of a poem or song lyric while you walk. Low or moderate-intensity exertion allows you to speak comfortably, without huffing and puffing or being out of breath. If you can't carry on a conversation or sing because you are short of breath or breathing too heavily, you are working too hard. Slow down!

Over time, you'll probably find that you can exert yourself harder or for longer durations and still be able to talk comfortably. That's an easy way to measure your progress.

Special Considerations

This method is not effective if you have asthma or another problem related to breathing. If so, you should use the perceived exertion or heart rate scales described here.

The Perceived Exertion Scale

The perceived exertion scale allows you to be more specific than the talk test in determining the intensity of your exercise. With perceived exertion, people score intensity based on how they feel.

To use this scale, you rate your effort on a scale of 1 to 10, which corresponds to exercise as feeling "very, very light" to "very, very hard." The numbers are identified on the scale below. For example, if you stated that the effort you were exerting was at the "hard" level, the corresponding number to this would be 8 or above on a scale of 10.

If you are a brand-new exerciser, have significant limitations or are older, you should begin walking at a "very light" level (2) or at most a "fairly light" level (3) of exertion for you. That would be a slow walk or stroll. Over time, gradually increase your exertion level to walk at a "moderate/somewhat hard" level (4-7).

Even if you are very fit, do not exercise at a level that is above 8 on the perceived exertion scale (what you would describe as "very hard"). At that point you are at increased risk for injury.

PERCEIVED EXERTION SCALE	
Numeric rating of your exertion	Verbal description of your exertion
0	Nothing at all (such as lying down)
1	Very, very light (practically nothing)
2	Very light
3	Fairly light
4	Moderate (still light but starting to work a little more)
5	Moderate (still comfortable but harder)
6	Moderate (getting to be somewhat hard)
7	Somewhat hard
8	Hard
9	Very hard
10	Very, very hard (couldn't do for more than a few seconds)

Heart Rate Scale

For most people, monitoring your intensity by taking your pulse and using the heart rate scale is the most accurate way to measure your aerobic intensity. By finding out what your target heart rate is you ensure that you are working at a safe and effective level for you.

Moderate aerobic intensity – the kind of walking that is recommended for health and fitness – should raise your heart rate into a range between 60 percent and 75 percent of your maximum heart rate. This range is called your target heart rate (THR) and is the recommended level for walking for most people with arthritis.

Be aware that maximum heart rate declines with age, so your safe THR gets lower as you get older. You can use the target heart rate scale and the outlined steps below to find your targeted heart rate.

TARGET HEART RATE SCALE (THR)				
Age	Max Heart Rate	One Minute Count		10-Second Count	
		60% of max	75% of max	60% of max	75% of max
20-24	200	120	150	20	25
25-29	195	117	146	19	24
30-34	190	114	142	19	24
35-39	185	111	139	18	23
40-44	180	108	135	18	22
45-49	175	105	131	17	22
50-54	170	102	127	17	21
55-59	165	99	124	16	21
60-64	160	96	120	16	20
65-69	155	93	116	15	19
70-74	150	90	112	15	19
75+	145	87	108	14	18

How To Take Your Pulse

You should measure your heart rate a few minutes into your exercise program to determine how much you are exerting yourself. To use the heart rate scale to monitor walking, you need to know how to take your pulse. You'll need a clock or watch with a second hand. Here are the steps for a 10-second heart rate count.

1. Take your pulse by placing the pads of your middle two or three fingers on your wrist below the base of your thumb. Do not use your thumb to take your pulse because it has its own pulse and will obstruct the counting of your actual pulse. You should be able to feel your blood pumping and the "thump" of your heart beating. (Some people take the pulse at the carotid artery in the neck. If you do this, be careful not to press too hard, which can cut or slow blood flow.)

2. Get your clock or watch ready and for 10 seconds count how many beats you feel. Begin your count with zero for the first beat you feel.

3. Multiply your number of heartbeats by 6 to find out how many times your heart is beating in one minute.

4. Your number should fall within the 60 percent to 75 percent range of numbers for your age level on the THR Scale. If your number is too high, you are exercising too intensely. Slow down. If your number is too low, and you feel OK, you can work harder.

5. Some people have trouble getting their heart rate up to the lower rate, particularly at first. Don't worry about that. As you become experienced and stronger, your heart rate will rise because you are exercising more vigorously.

Special Considerations

If you are pregnant or are taking blood pressure, heart or other medicines that affect your heart rate, this method will not be accurate. If you currently are using any medicines listed below, don't use the target heart rate scale; monitor your intensity by using the talk test or the rate of perceived exertion scale:

- alpha blockers

- beta blockers

- calcium channel blockers

- nitrates

- non-adrenergic peripheral vasodilators

- centrally acting or peripheral acting adrenergic inhibitors

- tricyclic antidepressants

- major tranquilizers

- cold medicines

- diet medicines

- bronchodilators

Measuring Your Fitness Level

Measuring your fitness level is easy. There are three good methods: measure how far you can walk during a set period of time; walk a specific distance and see how long it takes; or measure your heart rate for a certain amount of exertion (such as walking a period of time).

This provides you with a good gauge of your progress, especially if you do this at the beginning and ending point of a contract with yourself, as outlined in Chapter 2.

Equipment you'll need

- Watch with second hand or a stopwatch (to take pulse count and to measure time if you are walking a specific distance)

- Pedometer, car odometer or other form of measuring distance (to measure distance if you are walking for a designated amount of time)

- Pencil and paper to record time and/or pulse rate

- Comfortable walking shoes and clothing

Measuring may sound complicated, but it really isn't! Follow these steps:

1. Choose a length of time that you can walk without stopping – for example, 10 minutes.

Or, determine a distance that you *can* complete, no matter how long it would take – around the block 10 times, up to the corner and back, or whatever.

2. Find a smooth, level surface where you can measure your distance fairly accurately, such as a track, neighborhood streets or your local shopping mall. Try to avoid lots of stoplights and heavy traffic areas if you can. If you can't avoid these, that's OK. Just continue to march lightly in place while you wait for any delays.

3. Warm up and stretch, using the same warm up that you will do before each walking session (see Chapter 3).

4. Write down the time you start and the place you are starting. It is important that you try not to stop at any time during the test. If you are getting tired, slow down as much as you need to, even down to a very slow walk, but keep walking until you have completed your entire time or distance. If you do need to stop, that's fine – you'll now have a better idea of what is doable for you. Do your test on another day, and choose a better distance or time for you.

5. Once you've completed your predetermined walking time, note where you are (in front of the yellow house or at the corner of First and Elm). Keep moving slowly for a few minutes and then stretch to cool down.

If you are walking for a predetermined distance, note the time that you reached your stopping point.

Keep moving slowly for a few minutes and then stretch to cool down.

If you choose to use the heart rate scale, take your pulse for ten seconds before you start your cool down. Multiply by 6 or use the conversion chart on the scale above to determine your beats per minute. Then record your one-minute pulse rate.

6. If you walked for a designated amount of time (10 minutes, etc.), measure the distance you traveled during that time, either by using a pedometer, your car odometer, or counting the number of times you circled the track or mall. Note the distance on your contract or in your diary.

If you chose to walk for a set distance (around the block 10 times, etc.), record the time it took to walk your distance in minutes and seconds.

If you measured your heart rate, record it on your contract or in your diary.

That's it! At regular times during your plan – or at least at the end of the contract – take the fitness test following the above steps to track your progress. You probably will see that you can walk for a longer distance during your designated time. Alternatively, you may find you are able to complete the same distance in a shorter time.

Either way, that's a sign of improvement in your fitness level! If you don't see any change, that's OK. You may be at a level that is just right for you, and which you comfortably can continue.

Final Considerations

This entire book has been designed to help you develop the kind of walking program that is safe, effective and doable. It's a program that you'll be able to keep up for a lifetime of better health.

Review all of the chapters for suggestions concerning good exercise techniques and safety. Discuss any questions you have with your doctor or therapist. Always remember to move at your own pace. Progress slowly and gradually. Don't forget to keep your records. Do your best, challenge yourself if you can, but don't try to keep up with anyone else. Your *Walk With Ease* program is for you, to help you self-manage your arthritis and become healthier and fit!

Self-Check

❏ I know how to measure my walking intensity.

❏ I have a plan to measure my fitness level.

❏ I understand the importance of recognizing exercise limitations and safety considerations.

❏ I know I can keep up my walking program, regardless of obstacles.

Remember

When it comes to exercise, keep telling yourself, "I can do this!" It's only 30 minutes of walking a day, three to five days a week to make your joints, bones, muscles and heart more fit and healthier. That's just two to three hours out of the entire 168 hours in a week. For the remaining 165 hours in the week, you will feel better, experience less pain, have more energy, be stronger and have a brighter emotional outlook as a result of the time you've spent walking. Good luck!

Contracts and Diaries

***WALK WITH EASE* CONTRACT**

Name: _____

Dates: _____ to _____

The Plan:
To walk _____ days a week for _____ minutes a day,
broken into _____ sessions.

To include:
_____ Minutes warming up and stretching
_____ Minutes walking
_____ Minutes cooling down and stretching

I am sure I can complete this plan (circle):
0   1   2   3   4   5   6   7   8   9   10
(not at all sure)   (totally sure)

**When I complete this program, my reward to myself
will be:**

_____

_____

_____

How did I do?

_____

_____

_____

WALKING DIARY

Daily Record

For each day you walk, write down how long or how far you walked.

Week	S	M	T	W	T	F	S	Total
1								
2								
3								
4								
5								
6								
7								
8								
9								
10								

Starting Self-Test Measurement(s) (e.g., target heart rate check, rate of perceived exertion)

_____

_____

_____

Ending Self-Test Measurement(s)

_____

_____

_____

WALKING DIARY								
Daily Record								

For each day you walk, write down how long or how far you walked.

Week	S	M	T	W	T	F	S	Total
1								
2								
3								
4								
5								
6								
7								
8								
9								
10								

Starting Self-Test Measurement(s) (e.g., target heart rate check, rate of perceived exertion)

_____

_____

_____

Ending Self-Test Measurement(s)

_____

_____

_____

WALKING DIARY

Daily Record

For each day you walk, write down how long or how far you walked.

Week	S	M	T	W	T	F	S	Total
1								
2								
3								
4								
5								
6								
7								
8								
9								
10								

Starting Self-Test Measurement(s) (e.g., target heart rate check, rate of perceived exertion)

_____

_____

_____

Ending Self-Test Measurement(s)

_____

_____

_____

WALKING DIARY								
Daily Record								

For each day you walk, write down how long or how far you walked.

Week	S	M	T	W	T	F	S	Total
1								
2								
3								
4								
5								
6								
7								
8								
9								
10								

Starting Self-Test Measurement(s) (e.g., target heart rate check, rate of perceived exertion)

_____

_____

_____

Ending Self-Test Measurement(s)

_____

_____

_____

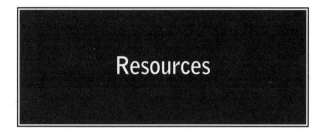

CHAPTER 7

Resources

About the Arthritis Foundation

For more than 50 years, the Arthritis Foundation has been the source for reliable information for the more than 43 million Americans with arthritis. It is the only national, voluntary health organization that works for all people affected by any of the more than 100 forms of arthritis or related conditions. Chapters nationwide help to support research, professional and community education programs, services for people with arthritis, government advocacy and fund-raising activities.

The mission of the Arthritis Foundation is to provide leadership in the prevention, control and cure of arthritis and related diseases. Public contributions and sales of books like this one enable the Arthritis Foundation to fulfill this mission, by helping to fund research, programs and services. The Arthritis Foundation has more than 150 chapters and branch offices all around the United States that provide support for people living with arthritis, including physician referrals, programs and activities, and useful information that helps people with arthritis lead healthier, more fulfilling lives. Arthritis doesn't have to prevent you from doing the activities you enjoy most. While research holds the key to future cures or preventions for arthritis, equally important is improving the quality of life for people with arthritis today.

To find the Arthritis Foundation chapter or branch office near your home, and to determine which of the following resources are available through your nearest chapter, call **800/283-7800** or log on to **www.arthritis.org**.

Arthritis Help Online

The Arthritis Foundation's interactive Web site, **www.arthritis.org**, provides a great deal of information and resources that are easy to access 24 hours a day from your home computer.

The site offers a confidential self-management guidance program called *Connect and Control,* where you can enter personal information about your health situation and receive a custom-made program for improving your diet, health, fitness and pain-management.

The Web site also helps you find your local chapter easily. Many Arthritis Foundation chapters have their own Web site pages that will inform you about activities in your community, as well as exciting opportunities to take part in fund-raising events, walks and marathons. In addition, you can read free material on **www.arthritis.org**, including in-depth feature stories from *Arthritis Today* magazine and news stories about new research, hot trends and thought-provoking issues related to arthritis prevention and treatment.

On the Arthritis Foundation Web site, you can talk to other people with arthritis through online message boards, ask questions about your condition and treatment, request free brochures and purchase books and videos to help you better manage your arthritis. The Arthritis Store contains information about the many books, brochures and exercise videos published by the Arthritis Foundation. You can also buy Arthritis Foundation books and videos by calling **800/207-8633**.

Arthritis Foundation Chapters – What They Offer You

If you have arthritis, your best source of information and support is your local Arthritis Foundation chapter. The staff at your nearest chapter or branch office has many resources to help you live a healthier, more fulfilling life with arthritis. If you are newly diagnosed with a form of arthritis, contact your chapter to find out what they have to offer you, including the following:

- **Brochures.** The Arthritis Foundation chapter nearest you will have an array of free, educational brochures on a wide variety of arthritis-related topics, from specific diseases, lifestyle challenges, current medications and more. All brochures are concise and easy to understand, and point you to other resources for managing your arthritis.

- **Physician Referral.** Most Arthritis Foundation chapters can give you a list of doctors in your area who specialize in the evaluation and treatment of arthritis and arthritis-related diseases.

- **Exercise Programs.** The Arthritis Foundation sponsors a number of exercise programs, both land- and water-based, that benefit beginners as well as exercise veterans. No matter what your ability, the Arthritis Foundation can help you get moving. These exercise programs are designed to accommodate people with arthritis and take your physical limitations into consideration.

- **Classes and Courses.** Formal group meetings help people with various forms of arthritis gain the knowledge, skills and confidence they need to actively manage their conditions. Courses focus on proper exercises, medications, relaxation techniques, pain management, dealing with depression, nutrition, alternative treatments and doctor-patient relations. **Call 800/283-7800 to find your nearest chapter or branch.**

- **Information Hotline.** The Arthritis Foundation – the expert on arthritis – is only a phone call away. Call toll-free at **800/283-7800** for automated information on arthritis 24 hours a day. Trained volunteers and staff are also available at your local Arthritis Foundation to answer your questions or send you a list of physicians in your area who specialize in arthritis. Also, choose from our more than 70 educational booklets on different types of arthritis, medications, disease management, self-help and more.

Arthritis Today

The Arthritis Foundation's award-winning magazine, *Arthritis Today*, brings you up-to-date and reliable information about the latest research and treatment options, diet and nutrition, tips for traveling and making your life with arthritis easier and more rewarding. Subscribe to six issues a year of this award-winning health magazine and find all the information you need to achieve a healthier, more active life with arthritis. Call **800/207-8633** for subscription information, or log on to **www.arthritis.org** and click on *Arthritis Today* to read more about *AT* online.

Books

In addition to *Walk With Ease,* the Arthritis Foundation publishes a number of books for people with arthritis and others seeking to create a healthier lifestyle. All Arthritis Foundation books are available by calling **800/207-8633**, or by logging on to **www.arthritis.org**, and selecting the Arthritis Store tab. The retail price and item number are included in the following descriptions of each book. Arthritis Foundation books are also sold in bookstores nationwide.

All Arthritis Foundation books are given a thorough medical review by leading physicians and health-care professionals, so you can be sure that you are receiving sound information about your health, fitness and arthritis management.

Books Available from the Arthritis Foundation:

The Arthritis Foundation's Guide to Managing Your Arthritis. This comprehensive, yet clear and easy-to-read book offers basic information about managing your arthritis. The book discusses the many types of arthritis, how your doctor will diagnose your condition, common drugs, surgical and alternative therapies for arthritis, and how you can treat symptoms and create an active, fulfilling life with arthritis. $24.95 / #835-245

The Arthritis Foundation's Guide to Good Living With Osteoarthritis

The Arthritis Foundation's Guide to Good Living With Rheumatoid Arthritis

The Arthritis Foundation's Guide to Good Living With Fibromyalgia

Get specific information about taking control of your condition in one of this series of books. Each book offers information on diagnosis, causes, drugs, surgical techniques, self-management strategies and alternative therapies. You'll find a handy guide to prescription and over-the-counter drugs for the particular disease, and easy exercises you can do to improve mobility and reduce pain.
$16.95 each
Osteoarthritis: #835-221
Rheumatoid Arthritis: #835-222
Fibromyalgia: #835-228

Tips for Good Living With Arthritis. You'll find more than 700 tips for making your daily activities easier and less painful in this handy guidebook. The book offers basic information about the most common types of arthritis, and what you can do to protect your joints as you go about your day.
$9.95 / #835-230

The Arthritis Foundation's Guide to Alternative Therapies. Yoga, glucosamine, kava kava, copper bracelets…You may be curious about the many alternative and complementary therapies touted for easing arthritis pain and other symptoms. Learn the truth behind the advertising and find the therapies that may work for you.
$24.95 / #835-220

Health Organizer: A Personal Health-Care Record. Spiral-bound and tabbed for convenient use, this organizer keeps all your medical and insurance records in one location and helps you track your symptoms with useful prompts.
$14.95 / #835-207

Toward Healthy Living: A Wellness Journal. Today's health experts recommend keeping a journal to express your feelings and monitor your arthritis or related condition. This beautifully designed, spiral-bound journal not only gives you space to collect your thoughts, but it contains areas to monitor you mood and pain levels. Plus, you'll discover words of wisdom shared by a variety of famous and "everyday" people who live with chronic illness. Take care of your mind as well as your body.
$14.95 / #835-205

Celebrate Life: New Attitudes for Living With Chronic Illness. Nurse, counselor, mother – and a woman with arthritis. Author Kathleen Lewis, RN, offers practical experience and guidelines for creating a fulfilling life with a chronic illness. Lewis explores diagnosis and medical treatment, dealing with family and friends, sexuality and finding the inner strength to celebrate your life despite your arthritis.
$12.95 / #835-219

Beyond Chaos: One Man's Journey Alongside his Chronically Ill Wife. Author and consultant Gregg Piburn offers a candid, revealing and inspiring look at being a spouse of a person with a chronic illness. Piburn examines his role as his wife,

Sherrie, dealt with fibromyalgia, including the struggle to find a diagnosis and the dramatic shifts in their relationship.
$14.95 / #835-214

Raising a Child with Arthritis: A Parent's Guide. Get reliable advice and information from the top pediatric health professionals in the nation. This is your essential guide to understanding and coping with the challenges of caring for a child with arthritis.
$14.95 / #835-209

Videotapes

People with Arthritis Can Exercise (PACE) Videos I & II. Designed to help you keep moving and stay active, PACE exercise programs consist of gentle routines led by golfer Jan Stephenson. Both PACE levels include stretching, strengthening and fitness exercises. Level II includes a longer endurance-building segment.
PACE Level I: $19.50 / #835-9010
PACE Level II: $19.50 / #835-9020

Pool Exercise Program (PEP). Participate in the Arthritis Foundation's famous Pool Exercise Program in the comfort of your home before you head to the pool. The PEP video features water exercises that will help you increase and maintain joint flexibility, strengthen and tone muscles, and increase endurance. All exercises are performed in water at chest level. No swimming skills are necessary.
$19.50 / #835-9030

Fibromyalgia Interval Training (FIT). Designed specifically to help people with fibromyalgia manage pain, stiffness and fatigue, this videotape demonstrates exercises that will keep you active. Learn about warm water exercises in both shallow and deep water, including warm-up, stretching, upper and lower body exercises, aerobics, strengthening, cool-down and relaxation techniques. $29.99 / #835-9040

Senderos para Vivir Mejor con la Artritis y condiciones afines. A Spanish-language video guide to achieving a better life with arthritis or related diseases, including stretching, breathing techniques, relaxation strategies and aerobic activity. $29.99 / #835-9051

Other Resources
Journal Articles
Arthritis Care and Research: Exercise and Arthritis Special Theme Issue, 7:167-236, 1994.

Coleman EA, Buchner DM, et al. The relationship of joint symptoms with exercise performance in older adults. *J Amer Geriat Soc 44:14-21, 1996.*

Ettinger WH, Afable RF. Physical disability from knee arthritis: the role of exercise as an intervention. *Med Sci Sport Exercise* 26:1435-1440, 1994.

Ettinger WH, Burns R, et al. A randomized trial comparing aerobic exercise and resistance exercise with a health education program in older adults with knee arthritis: The fitness arthritis and seniors trial (FAST). *JAMA*. 227: 25-31, 1997.

Harkcom TA, Lampman RM, Banwell BF, Castor CW. Therapeutic value of graded aerobic exercise training in rheumatoid arthritis. *Arthritis Rheum* 28:32-39, 1985.

Kovar PA, Allegrante JP, et al. Supervised fitness walking in patients with osteoarthritis of the knee. *Ann Intern Med* 116:529-534, 1992.

Lorig K, Holman H. Arthritis self-management studies: A twelve year review. *Health Education Quarterly* 20: 17-28, 1993.

Minor MA. Physical activity and management of arthritis. *Ann Behav Med* 13:117-124, 1990.

Minor MA, Hewett JE, et al. Efficacy on physical conditioning exercise in patients with rheumatoid arthritis and osteoarthritis. *Arthritis Rheum* 32:1396-1405, 1989.

Minor MA, Sanford MK. Physical interventions in the management of pain in arthritis. *Arthritis Care Res* 6:197-206, 1993.

Perlman SG, Connell KJ, et al. Dance-based aerobic exercise for rheumatoid arthritis. *Arthritis Care Res* 3:29-35, 1990.

Rippe JM, Ward A, Porcari JP, Freedson PS. Walking for health and fitness. JAMA 259:2720-2724, 1988.

Appendix: Exercises To Stretch and Strengthen Your Muscles

Stretches To Do Before and After You Walk

After you have warmed up (be sure to warm up by slowly walking or marching in place for 3 to 5 minutes first), do each of theses stretches. You don't want to stretch your muscles when they're cold. Hold each stretch for 20 to 30 seconds.

After your cool-down routine, repeat each of the stretches. Hold each stretch for 30 to 45 seconds.

Hints:

- Stretch just until you feel tension and then hold the stretch in that place.
- When you stretch, do not bounce. Make sure you stretch gently and smoothly.
- Be sure to do each stretch on both right and left sides.
- Breathe naturally as you hold the stretches. Don't hold your breath.

Upper Calf and Hip

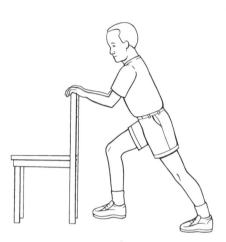

- Lean against a wall, tree or chair for support, and place one foot back. Keep toes facing forward.

- Bend the knee of the front leg, bringing it directly over the toes as you press hips forward. Keep head up and spine straight.

- Press the heel of the back foot into the floor.

- Hold for 20 to 30 seconds during warm-up or 30 to 45 seconds after cool down.

Lower Calf and Achilles Tendon

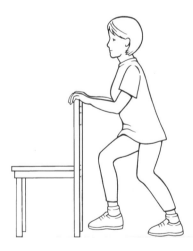

- Stay in Upper Calf stretch position, but move the back leg in slightly, toward the front leg.

- Bend the back knee and keep the heel of that foot pressed into the floor.

- Hold for 20 to 30 seconds during the warm-up or 30 to 45 seconds after cool down.

Illustrations by Kathryn Born

Side and Arm Stretch

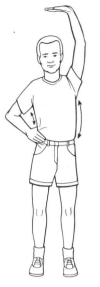

- Stand with your feet 18 inches apart, hips centered.

- Raise one arm out to your side and over your head, palm pointing inward.

- Stand straight, or bend just a few inches. Feel the stretch in your side.

- Repeat with the other arm raised.

Strengthening Exercises for Walking

Do these exercises two to three times each week to help strengthen the muscles and joints that are used when you walk.

Hints:

- Start off doing no more than five repetitions of each exercise.
- Gradually increase to no more than 10 repetitions of each.
- Be sure to do each exercise with both right and left sides.
- Go slowly and do each movement with control.
- Breathe naturally. Do not hold your breath!
- If you have increased pain that lasts for more than two hours after exercising, next time do fewer repetitions.

Quadriceps Lifts

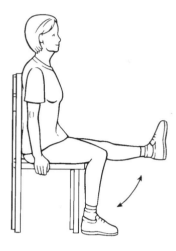

- Sitting in a chair, straighten the knee by tightening up the muscle on top of your thigh.

- Hold your knee as straight as possible. As your knee strengthens, see if you can build up to holding your leg out for 30 seconds. If straightening your knee from a fully bent position is uncomfortable, start with your foot resting on a low stool, as shown.

- Repeat several times.

- Do with other leg.

Ready to Go

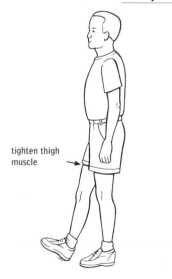

tighten thigh muscle →

- Stand with one foot slightly in front of the other, heel of the forward leg on the ground, and toes off the ground (as if you are going to take a step).

- Straighten and tighten the knee of the forward leg by tensing the muscles on the front of the thigh.

- Hold for a count of five. Relax. Repeat several times.

- Do with other leg.

Down and Ups

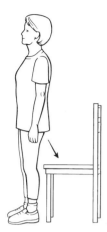 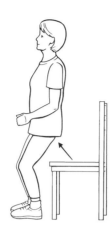

- Standing in front of a chair with arms at your sides, slowly bend your hips and knees as if you were going to sit down.

- Lower yourself only halfway, then straighten your hips and knees to stand back up again. Do not use your hands to help.

- Repeat several times.

Ankle Rotations

- Sit in a straight-backed chair with your feet bare.

- With your heels on the ground, slowly circle your ankles to the right and then to the left. Go as far in each direction as you can.

Foot Raises

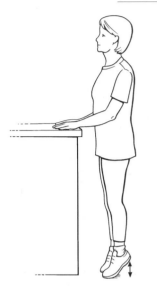

- Hold on to a counter or table for support

- Rise up on your tiptoes. Hold for five seconds.

- Lower slowly.

- Repeat several times.

  NOTE: How high you go is not as important as keeping your balance and controlling your ankles. It is easier to do both legs at the same time. If your feet are too sore, wear shoes or do it while sitting down.

Hip Flexor Stretch

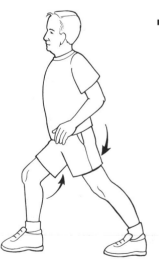

- Place your right foot in front of your left foot. Tuck your buttocks tightly under your hips while you contract your abdominal (stomach) muscles. You will feel a stretch on the front of your left hip and upper thigh. Hold for a few seconds. Switch feet and repeat.

Standing Hamstring Stretch

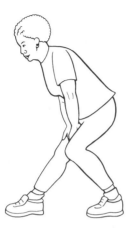

- Place your right foot in front of your left foot. Lean forward. Support your hands on the top of your left thigh. Gently drop your hips and buttocks backward until you feel mild tension on the back of your right thigh. Don't "lock" your right knee. Hold for a few seconds, then repeat placing the left foot forward.

Raised Leg Hamstring Stretch

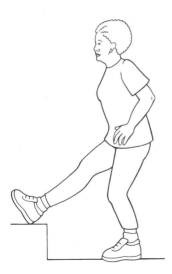

- Place your right leg on a slightly raised surface, like a step in your house or the curb outside. Keep your hips facing forward. Slowly bend your left knee until you feel a mild tension or stretch on the back of your right thigh. Hold for a few seconds. Repeat using the other leg.

Standing Quadriceps Stretch

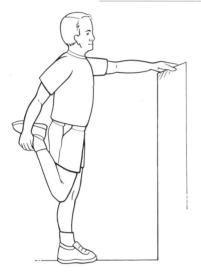

■ Hold on to a supportive railing, wall or tall object with your left hand. Grasp your right foot with your right hand. Gently pull your right heel toward your buttocks. Hold for a few seconds. Repeat using the left leg.

NOTE: Don't arch your back! Make sure your knee points straight down when you bend your leg with both knees as close together as possible. Don't ''lock'' the knee of your straight, supporting leg.

Toe Raises Stretch

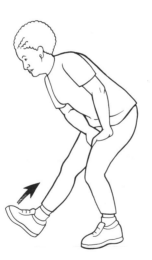

■ Put your body in the same position as you did to begin the standing hamstring stretch. Lift your right toes. Hold for a few seconds. Repeat using the other foot.

Crossover Stretch

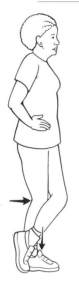

■ Cross your left shin and foot over your right shin and foot. Curl up your left toes so that the top of your left shoe (or the shoelaces) is pointing downward. Gently press your right knee into your left calf muscle until you feel a mild stretch or tension in your left shin. Hold for a few seconds. Repeat by crossing the right leg over the left leg.

Head Circle Neck Stretch

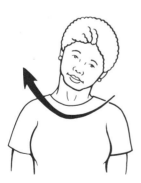

■ Slowly move your head in a circular motion from your left shoulder to your right shoulder. Reverse the motion and repeat several times.

NOTE: Don't try to make a circle leaning backward, as this motion can place unnecessary strain on the cervical spine.

Head Tilt Stretch

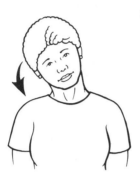

- Gently tilt your head to the right, moving your right ear downward toward your right shoulder. Hold for a few seconds. Repeat using the left side.

Head Rotation Stretch

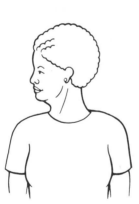

- Gently rotate your head to the right, so that you are looking over your right shoulder. Hold for a few seconds. Repeat by rotating your head to the left side.

Shoulder Circle Stretch

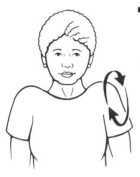

■ Make circles with both of your shoulders, moving them in a backward circle eight times.

Overarm Shoulder Press Stretch

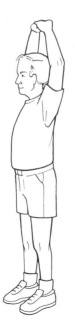

■ Lift your arms and clasp your hands together above your head. Make sure your elbows are slightly bent. Slowly push your arms backward. Hold for a few seconds.

Underarm Shoulder Press Stretch

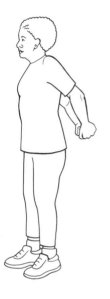

- Reach your arms back behind you and clasp your hands together behind your back. Make sure your elbows are slightly bent. Slowly raise your arms a bit. Hold for a few seconds.

Notes

Notes

Notes

Get the Most Out of Life!

ONLY
$24.95

TO ORDER, VISIT
www.arthritis.org
or Call Toll Free:
1-800-207-8633
(M-F 8 a.m. - 5 p.m EST)

Create A More Healthy, Fulfilling Future.

The Arthritis Foundation's new **Guide to Managing Your Arthritis** gives you all the information you need to make the most of every day. This easy-to-understand book helps you manage pain, reduce stress, work with your health-care team and make sense of drugs, surgery and supplements. You'll learn simple exercises to help you ease stiffness and feel more mobile. Whether you are new to arthritis or have lived with it for years, this book has life-enhancing strategies for you.

Get the tools you need to create a more active, fulfilling life!

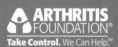

BKADWWE1

Get Moving Again!

ARTHRITIS FOUNDATION®
Take Control. We Can Help.™

An Arthritis Foundation Exercise Program

VHS

PACE™

LEVEL 1

People with Arthritis **Can** Exercise

A gentle exercise program with champion golfer Jan Stephenson— made for people with arthritis, by people who know and care about arthritis

Get moving again with this great video!

People with Arthritis Can Exercise (PACE) from the Arthritis Foundation gets "two thumbs up" from viewers! You'll work out to a gentle exercise program hosted by champion golfer Jan Stephenson. This 30-minute video promises to get you moving again and to help you regain the ability to do everyday activities!

You can exercise with PACE!

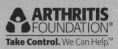

ARTHRITIS FOUNDATION®
Take Control. We Can Help.™

BKWWE2